'This book centres on seminal research undertaken to examine the complex, multifactorial, organisational, professional and interpersonal elements that shape and influence midwives' behaviour, role, expectations and clinical work. It offers a unique and poignant insight into the tensions, challenges and opportunities that many working midwives encounter as they navigate their way through an increasing polarisation between the alignment of a professional mandate anchored in a social model of enablement and advocacy for women and their families and employer expectations and constraints. A shortfall of skilled midwives is not unique to the UK. However, this is not occurring solely because of retirement; attrition is a major issue, be it midwives switching to work part-time or leaving midwifery because they do not receive the support, respect or resources to enable them to provide personalised skilled care. This research presents an important resource for all maternity stakeholders to consider and reflect upon when shaping humane, dynamic, supporting organisations that enable midwives to thrive'.

Dr Ethel Burns, *Senior Lecturer Midwifery,*
Oxford Brookes University

'This is such an important book addressing the ethical, cultural, and political challenges faced by midwives supporting physiological birth choices and women navigating maternity care in the current climate. The author is extremely knowledgeable on the field of personalised care and the complexities associated with its implementation in the real world. This is an essential book to understand how we got here in the first place and how we can move on, putting women and birthing people at the helm and facilitate whatever choice they make, in any setting they choose'.

Lia Brigante, *Midwife, RM, MSc*

'Claire Feeley's book comes at a critical time for midwifery. Centring the ethical concept of bodily autonomy, so intrinsic to midwifery practice, she identifies the tensions that arise for midwives, who are philosophically bound to be 'with-woman', when women make decisions that do not comply with recommended guidelines. That such a book needed to be written is already an indictment of maternity systems worldwide and their inability to provide individualised care. As reports of obstetric violence and birth trauma rise, this book provides an important contribution in its incisive discussion of the current pressures, but its real effect is in the offering of a solution – where midwives' professional responsibility to provide safe care can comfortably co-exist with women's choices, regardless of what that choice might be. A must-read for anyone interested in the culture, ethics, or practice of childbirth'.

Dr Elizabeth Newnham, *Senior Lecturer,*
University of Newcastle, Australia

'I propose that all those with an interest in maternity services should read and be guided by the findings and proposals in this book. We must learn from what works – meeting the needs and facilitating choice is possible when there is a culture of mutual respect, support and compassionate leadership. The text offers evidence-based practical solutions in an engaging and clear format – an absolute gem and gives me hope for the future'.

Sheena Byrom, *OBE, Midwife, Co-Founder*
ALL4Maternity

'Just finished reading your book, it is so good, so important, and so well written! I have felt rather despondent about midwifery and maternity services in the UK since I returned from practicing in New Zealand in 2012, it captures much of what I have been concerned about and I realise that part of me had 'given up the fight', as it has felt too big a challenge. But, reading this reminds me that it is too important to give up on… Congratulations on this work, thank you for articulating it so well'.

Dr Tomasina Stacey, *Midwife, Senior Lecturer*
King's College London

'This timely and articulate book urges us to think more deeply about the socio-cultural and political influences that shape midwives' practice and the care that they are able to offer to birthing women and people. Drawing on her original feminist narrative inquiry research, Claire Feeley vividly describes how UK midwives responded to women's requests for 'out of guidelines' birth choices and explores what can be learned from their responses. Using midwives' first-hand accounts of the challenges and enablers they experienced, a compelling argument is created: that compassionate leadership, trust in staff ability and in maternal autonomy are critical for high quality, respectful and culturally safe maternity services. An essential and thought-provoking read for everyone wanting to understand current debates in maternity care'.

Billie Hunter, *CBE, FRCM PhD, BNurs, RM, RN*
Emerita Professor. Cardiff University

'Claires passion for supporting physiological birth is infectious and her work incorporates a holistic approach to midwifery care. This book will provide the evidence base for midwives in practice to centre the needs and wishes of women and enable them to support physiology and individualised care'.

Cheryl Samuels, *'Holistic Midwife' and Lecturer, University*
of Suffolk

'This brilliant book is commanding and provocative in its argument for a truly equitable maternity service. From the vantage point of how midwives support physiological birth, Claire Feeley makes visible fundamental tensions in maternity care concerning birthing women and peoples' choices. Feeley's assessment of why 'out of guidelines' birth choices have come to be viewed as so problematic provides a comprehensive and considered account of the socio-cultural-political landscape of present-day services where medicalisation, standardisation, risk, governance, and litigation issues are the norm. Drawing on the views and experiences of midwives employed in the UK's National Health Service, this book shines a light on the barriers women and birthing people can face when asserting their autonomy, and also why midwives leave. Feeley is visionary in her conception of collective responsibility and the centrality of organisational culture and system-wide solutions towards more equitable maternity services. This book is essential reading'.

Dr Carol Kingdon, *Reader in Medical Sociology,*
University of Central Lancashire, and Hon. Research Associate,
University of Liverpool and Liverpool Women's NHS
Foundation Trust

SUPPORTING PHYSIOLOGICAL BIRTH CHOICES IN MIDWIFERY PRACTICE

Highlighting the experiences of midwives who provide care to women opting outside of guidelines in the pursuit of physiological birth, Claire Feeley looks at the impact on midwives themselves, and explores how teams and organisations support or discourage women's birth choices.

This book investigates the processes, experiences and sociocultural-political influences upon midwives who support women's alternative birthing choice and argues for a shift in perspective from notions of an individual's professional responsibility to deliver woman-centred care, to a broader, collective responsibility. The book begins by contextualising the importance of quality midwifery care with an exploration of the current debates to demonstrate how hegemonic birth discourse and maternity practices have detrimentally affected physiological birth rates, and the wellbeing of women who opt outside of maternity guidelines. It provides real life examples of how midwives can facilitate a range of birthing decisions within mainstream midwifery services. Moreover, an exploration of midwives' experiences of delivering such care is presented, revealing deeply polarised accounts from moral injury to job fulfilment. The polarised accounts are then presented within a new model to explore how a midwife's socio-political working context can significantly mediate or exacerbate the vulnerability, conflict and stigmatisation that they may experience as a result of supporting alternative birth choices. Finally, this book explores the implications of the findings, looking at how team and organisational culture can be developed to better support women and midwives, making recommendations for a systems approach to improving maternity services.

Discussing the invisible nature of midwifery work, what it means to deliver woman-centred care, and the challenges and benefits of doing so, this is a thought-provoking read for all midwives and future midwives. It is also an important contribution to interprofessional concerns around workforce development, sustainability, moral distress and compassion in health and social care.

Claire Feeley is a clinical midwife and researcher with over 13 years' experience in maternal, perinatal and infant health. Formerly the editor-in-chief of *The Practising Midwife*, Dr Feeley is now a lecturer and researcher at King's College London.

SUPPORTING PHYSIOLOGICAL BIRTH CHOICES IN MIDWIFERY PRACTICE

The Role of Workplace Culture, Politics and Ethics

Claire Feeley

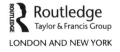

LONDON AND NEW YORK

Cover image: © Getty Images

First published 2023
by Routledge
4 Park Square, Milton Park, Abingdon, Oxon OX14 4RN

and by Routledge
605 Third Avenue, New York, NY 10158

Routledge is an imprint of the Taylor & Francis Group, an informa business

© 2023 Claire Feeley

British Library Cataloguing-in-Publication Data
A catalogue record for this book is available from the British Library

ISBN: 978-1-032-20831-2 (hbk)
ISBN: 978-1-032-20827-5 (pbk)
ISBN: 978-1-003-26544-3 (ebk)

DOI: 10.4324/9781003265443

Typeset in Bembo
by codeMantra

For James, my darling son, what a wild ride we have had so far! Thank you for being you, I love you.

CONTENTS

FIGURES

TABLES

FOREWORD

I have been lucky to be part of Claire's journey over the last decade – first, as her master's dissertation supervisor where she explored women's reasons for freebirthing and then as the Director of Studies for her PhD, which is the focus here. This book is centred on choice for a specific type of birth – a vaginal physiological birth. Overall, choice is a contested term, as, on the one hand, it suggests equity in that there are options that all can choose from, people have free choice to decide their preferred option and for what they choose to be a viable option. However, often the reality in a maternity context, choices that women and birthing people can make are inexplicably linked to risk, fear and litigation. As soon as there is a potential for perceived risk, then 'choices' can become rhetorical. In this book, Claire questions the constructs of the risk discourse and 'guideline-centred care' as an enforcement tool– this is whereby women's choices can be shaped by standardisation, institutionalisation and risk. While bound within a tautology of guidelines needing to be used as guidelines, Claire's research stems from the knowledge that these are often used as clinical 'rules' to restrict women and birthing peoples' bodily autonomy in how and where they give birth. This can be particularly apparent for a physiological birth, particularly when the birth is perceived as having higher risks, and where healthcare professionals have potentially less input and control over what happens.

While risk-based care has been the focus of a wealth of literature, Claire's aim was to explore a unique perspective of how midwives and maternity structures enable choice for a physiological birth when the women's and birthing people's history or physiological signs indicate otherwise – referred to as an 'out of guidelines' birth or, as Claire's refers, an alternative physiological birth. She also focused her research on midwives who were employed by the NHS to understand how choice can be enabled when operating within its arguably more rigid and institutional-based confines. Claire's work beautifully captures stories from

45 midwives who work across the UK and uses a theoretical model to depict the polarised accounts of how midwives can (or are restricted to) support an alternative physiological birth. At one end of the continuum, she describes emotive accounts of midwives who face stigma, and moral distress when deviating from 'usual care' to occasions of midwives having to 'bend the rules' to operate outside of expected norms, through to accounts of mutually supportive and multidisciplinary collaboration when more authentic forms of choice are enacted. This is a book that speaks of hope, resilience and courage, and provides practical strategies and approaches from an individual, team and organisational perspective. It reflects a salutogenic approach that illuminates not only the challenges that can be faced but also the occasions of when, how and by whom alternative physiological birth choices can be enabled. Giving birth is one of the most significant and important life transitions – this book emulates the values of essential maternity care by offering ways to enable and optimise safe and personalised care, and to ensure the physical and psychological wellbeing of all.

Professor Gill Thomson, University of Central Lancashire

There has been significant debate about the current state of midwifery around the world. Staffing shortages, moral distress and a rising exodus of staff characterise the debate. Reasons proposed for staff attrition have included poor life-work balance, overwork, incapacity to do the kind of midwifery midwives want to do, or to ensure safety for women, birthing people and babies, neoliberalist consumerism, individualism and/or technocracy. However, in all this theoretical debate, the voice of midwives themselves has been relatively silent.

In this book, Claire Feeley has unpacked some of the most deeply felt stories of midwives working at the edges of standard maternity care through the lens of so-called 'out of guidelines' situations. This focus provides new insights into all the theories listed above, through the perspective of 'emotionality' and psychological safety. The stories of the included midwives illustrate the hypocrisy of maternity systems that, rhetorically, claim to promote 'women-centred care' but that routinely expect midwives to 'talk women into' going along with whatever the local guidelines stipulate. While being rigorous and comprehensive, the text also conveys the everyday soul-damaging grind of trying to uphold values of personalisation and choice, while being regularly gainsaid or even ostracised by colleagues. Some of the accounts of moral distress and even of moral injury are heart-breaking. They deserve to be heard alongside the accounts of women and families whose lives are devastated by loss and harm, as equal casualties of a system that seems to be unable to acknowledge that it does not always enable its staff to enact its own rhetoric of woman-centred care.

However, alongside this clear-eyed critique of the harm caused by systems that act in bad faith, Claire also provides a joyous picture of how it is for those who are supported in the 'everyday enactment' of out of guidelines care. The stories of mutual collegiate support, care, true woman-centred care and autonomy, trust and positive relationships are polar opposites of the harrowing accounts in previous chapters. There is a sense of lightness and joy in the writing, and of an emotional burden lifted – indeed of it never having been there in the first place. As Claire notes, this is the context in which midwives stay, women, birthing people and partners have safe and positive birth experiences (no matter how their baby is born) and there is a constant reservoir of hope and delight that underpins positive resilience. The critical question is – how do we move from blame, grief, fear and broken relationships in the everyday work of midwives towards joy, delight and physical, emotional and psychological safety for all involved? This book is an important and highly readable account of how this can and should happen – and urgently, if the safety and wellbeing of ALL women and babies is to be safeguarded into the future. As Claire says:

> Unburdened by conflict, a lessened mental and emotional load allowed the midwives to not only get on with the job, but to flourish; experiencing joy through relational care offered reciprocal gains, meaning-making and personal affect. These experiences of joy, awe and wonder are a source of resilience and likely contributing factors to why midwives stay.

Professor Soo Downe, University of Central Lancashire

PREFACE

A 'normal' physiological birth is one that starts spontaneously, progresses without incident nor requires medical intervention and ends in a spontaneous birth where the mother and baby are both well. Qualifying as a midwife in 2011, the term 'normal' birth was typical vernacular to describe these types of births and did not face the level of scrutiny or contention as the term does today – in the UK at least. While the rate of 'normal' physiological births had been steadily declining and inter/intra-professional and public opinions were divided as to what mode of birth was 'best' (as they continue to be), the terminology and concept of physiological birth were not particularly contentious. Today, the landscape has radically changed with 'normal' birth (spontaneous labour and birth) a site for significant tension and conflict with sharp polarisation and deepening divides. For birthing women and people who were failed by maternity services and did not get the medical care they wanted, such as access to pharmacological pain relief or caesarean sections, those situations have caused significant distress and trauma. Equally, there are birthing women and people denied access to the care of their choosing, such as homebirths, birth centres, birthing pools, etc., or who have felt coerced into accepting medical interventions they did not want. These situations also cause significant distress and trauma. For birth choices at either end of the continuum, the common sense and humanised approach would be to support and facilitate all births aligned with individual women's needs. Yet, this seems to be an enormous challenge in the UK maternity system.

This book is about physiological birth, specifically the choices women have actively made which sit 'outside' of maternity guidelines or recommendations (I call alternative physiological birth choices). These choices include a vast array of decisions from those with pre-existing medical disorders seeking midwifery-led care (home/birth centre) or perhaps those preferring hospital but do not want specific routine medical care or interventions, to those with healthy 'low risk' pregnancies declining aspects of care (and everything in between). Given the immense scrutiny physiological birth faces, decisions outside of the guidelines especially challenge the current rhetoric around maternal bodily autonomy, thus warranted further investigation. The topic was borne out of a combination of my own birth experience, clinical experience and previous research with women preferring to opt outside of maternity care altogether, to freebirth, as maternity services could not or would not meet their needs. Conducting those interviews was heart-wrenching and awe-inspiring influencing my research journey. I was frustrated and angry on their behalf, the maternity services did not support their decisions. The women's initial decisions, wants and needs were not radical or particularly taxing for a competent maternity professional, yet these women faced obstacles and barriers and most experienced some level of trauma.

It was knowing that midwives (and obstetricians) elsewhere did have the skills, competency and confidence to facilitate a wide range of physiological births (complex or otherwise) that informed my research direction. Birth (or maternity care) trauma is hugely important, but going upstream and minimising its occurrence in the first place was compelling. Evidence now points us to caregiving as a key modifiable risk factor for birth (maternity care) trauma where acts of compassionate, respectful and dignified care safeguard and mitigate against such trauma – this includes the proactive support and facilitation of birthing choices. Therefore, I wanted to learn from those midwives who were managing to provide physiological birth care deemed 'outside of the guidelines' and while in NHS practice. Focusing on the midwives' caregiving was an opportunity to learn from the primary/lead carer for childbearing people in the UK whose skillset should be optimising physiological processes. Moreover, midwives are typically positioned as the mediators, arbitrators or gatekeepers for birth choices so researching their practice would illuminate what could be achieved and a way to explore the tensions existing around physiological birth. This book reflects my PhD work that recruited 45 NHS midwives self-defined as willingly supportive of these birth choices. Using three different analyses three different research questions were asked and answered, how the midwives provided clinical care, their experiences of doing so and the sociocultural-political workplace influence on their practice. Broadly, the findings demonstrated the midwives' workplace context – the culture, politics and ethical values played a significant role in their ability to support women's alternative physiological birthing choices. Resonating with my freebirthing study, this book includes heart-breaking and awe-inspiring accounts as the midwives navigated the maternity system to meet the needs of those in their care.

This work has not been without its challenges or difficulties, for life does not stop for research (or clinical work for that matter), but it has been a joy and privilege to research with the 45 midwives in this study. They gave up their precious time to contribute to the study and the wider evidence base, some in the most perilous of circumstances. It is a known feature of midwifery practice that the art is passed down orally through storytelling, and these midwives did not disappoint. I personally and professionally learnt so much from listening to their vast array of experiences. I was moved by their steadfast commitment to the women in their care and the degree of vulnerability they shared. Sharing these stories with the wider maternity community has also been a privilege; connecting to numerous audiences nationally and internationally a strong resonance with the findings has been evident. With thanks to the study participants who articulated the hidden, unseen, ineffable qualities of meaningful midwifery care, which has connected with these audiences.

Conducting this research was not a solo effort, and I have heartfelt gratitude for my patient supervisors, Prof Gill Thomson and Prof Soo Downe. Dr Carol Kingdon, Dr Stephanie Heys, Dr Louise Hunt and Dr Naoimh McMahon all provided valuable support during the PhD itself and of course, since then. A big thank you to those who have supported this work in different ways, too many to mention but a shout out to Anna and Sheena Byrom and The Practising Midwife for the opportunities you have given me along the way. Also, I am so grateful to the RCM, ARM and Birthrights who supported this work by advertising the study; with their wide reach, I was able to recruit a fantastic range of midwives from across the UK. I also owe Dr Jane Carpenter a huge thank you as it was Jane's introduction which led to this work in a monograph format. Thanks are also due to the team at Routledge who have been so helpful and supportive throughout this process. And of course, my friends and family who have had to put up with yet another writing marathon – thank you!

Finally, a huge thank you to 'my' midwives, Sandy Sinclair and Gemma Jones. Whether they realised it or not, their 'practising outside of the box' facilitated a much wanted joyful and empowering birth which was life-changing in every which way. I owe you so much.

Claire Feeley, UK.

Sections of this book were originally published in journal articles, listed below. However, changes have been made for the purposes of this book.

Chapter 3

Feeley, C., Thomson, G., Downe, S. (2020) Understanding how NHS midwives facilitate women's alternative birthing choices: Findings from a feminist pragmatist study. *PLOS ONE* 15(11), e0242508. https://doi.org/10.1371/journal.pone.0242508

Chapters 4 and 5

Feeley, C., Thomson, G., Downe. S. (2021) 'Stories of distress versus fulfilment': A narrative inquiry of midwives' experiences supporting alternative birth choices in the UK National Health Service. *Women and Birth*, 35(5), e446–e55. https://doi.org/10.1016/j.wombi.2021.11.003

Other publications associated with the study

Feeley, C., Thomson, G., & Downe S (2019). Caring for women making unconventional birth choices: A meta-synthesis exploring the views, attitudes, and experiences of midwives. *Midwifery*, 72, 50–59.

Feeley, C. (2022) The ASSET model: What midwives need to support alternative physiological births (outwith guidelines). *The Practising Midwife*, 25(2), 26–30.

GLOSSARY

Alternative institutionalised birth settings   either type of midwifery-led birth centres; AMU: adjoined birth centred (within hospital grounds) or FMU: free standing birth centre (independent of hospital).

Augmentation of labour   artificial methods to speed up labour.

Band   the pay scale that operates within the NHS for nurses and midwives, normally ranges from Band 5 (newly qualified midwife) to Band 8 a-c (Consultant Midwife or Head of Midwifery or Director of Midwifery)

Breech   baby is bottom first in the womb.

Caesarean section   surgical birth via the abdomen.

Caseloading   women who are looked after by one midwife throughout the childbearing continuum (with minor exceptions such as sick or holiday leave).

Continuity of carer   where women are looked after by the same midwife within small team of midwives throughout the childbirth continuum.

Continuous electronic fetal monitoring   a machine that is used to monitor the baby's heartrate throughout labour using a doppler positioned on the mother's abdomen which is attached to the machine (also see telemetry).

Coordinator/shift lead   a senior midwife on labour ward/delivery suite who is in charge of the whole ward.

Core midwife   a midwife that has a permanent job in one particular area i.e. labour ward/delivery suite or postnatal ward or antenatal clinic.

Episiotomy   a surgical cut to the perineum to aid delivery of the baby, commonly used in instrumental births, historically overused and can cause increased levels of perineal damage.

Fragmented care model   where women are seen by different (usually unknown) caregivers (midwives or doctors) throughout the childbearing continuum.

Grand-multipara   a woman who has had over 5 births (also see multiparous).

Group B Streptococcus a transient bacterial infection that can occur in approximately 20% of women.

Hypothyroidism underactive thyroid.

Induction of labour artificial method to initiate labour.

Instrumental births the use of forceps or ventouse to deliver the baby.

Integrated models where midwives offer continuity of care but work across homebirth and birth centre settings.

Intermittent monitoring/auscultation listening to the baby's heart rate at recurrent times throughout the first and second stage of labour; however, this is not continuous. It is carried out using either a pinard or a handheld doppler.

Intrapartum care caring for women during the labour and birthing period.

Meconium the faeces of an in-utero infant (whether presence of meconium is deemed significant depends upon gestation, stage of labour, presentation of baby and fetal heart sounds).

Multiparous a woman who has given birth more than once (also see grand-multipara).

Multi-professional team wider team that the midwife works with, could include obstetricians, paediatricians, specialist doctors, management and GPs.

Pre-eclampsia toxaemia a potentially life-threatening disorder of pregnancy, only resolved by birth.

Polyhydramnios excessive amniotic fluid in the amniotic sac.

Post-dates/post-term pregnancy beyond 40 weeks

Post-partum haemorrhage excessive bleeding after birth.

Prolonged slower than expected progress of particular stage of labour (also see stalled).

Rotational midwife midwife who works on a rotational basis to different departments i.e. labour ward/delivery suite, postnatal ward, antenatal clinic, community.

Shoulder dystocia during birth, the baby's shoulders get stuck and require active intervention to free them - is life threatening if not resolved.

Stalled labour slower than expected progress of particular stage of labour (also see prolonged).

Third degree tear laceration is a tear in the vaginal tissue, perineal skin and perineal muscles that extend into the anal sphincter.

Traditional community settings relates to midwives working in the community, often with their own caseload of antenatal women and work on calls for homebirths. However, they do not offer continuity of carer so are likely to provide intrapartum care for women they have not met.

Transfer moving from homebirth or birth centre to hospital, normally associated with complications of labour or during the immediate post-partum period.

Uterine rupture An obstetric emergency where both maternal and fetal lives are at significant risk as the uterus has ruptured.

Vaginal examination an internal examination to assess cervical changes.

Telemetry a wireless CEFM.

1

INTRODUCTION

This chapter sets the scene and introduces the research that focused on NHS midwives facilitating 'out of guidelines' physiological birth choices (or as I refer to, alternative physiological birth choices). Such decisions should, in theory, be upheld within UK policy, guidelines and legislation; however, evidence suggests birthing women and people can face moralistic opposition and restricted access to care of their choosing. Therefore, bodily autonomy for some women is largely rhetorical. Echoing wider, international literature, these issues are not unique to the UK. However, within the context of a strong midwifery-led workforce, integrated maternity and neonatal service infrastructure that supports birth in all settings and collaborative working with medical professionals, it is a curious situation in which physiological births outside of guidelines are a site for tension. Furthermore, midwives supporting these birth choices too can experience conflict when delivering their care. However, less was known regarding the experiences of midwives employed by the NHS, who willingly facilitated alternative physiological birth care. As a significant gap in the evidence base, this study sought to fill it to provide practice-based research that could be used to improve women's access to and experiences of alternative physiological birth care. Accordingly, this chapter first provides a discussion regarding the contemporary international evidence and debates surrounding childbirth and midwifery-led care. Second, 'alternative physiological births' are explained and the justification for exploring these issues from the midwives' perspectives is provided. Finally, an overview of the research is presented, providing insights into the participants, data collection and analysis to contextualise the rest of the book.

Childbirth and midwifery: Setting the scene

Birth is a biopsychosocial-cultural event with different layers of meaning depending on whose perspective. How birth is viewed, experienced and facilitated are

DOI: 10.4324/9781003265443-1

influenced by sociocultural-political contexts. Midwives, as the lead professionals of childbearing women (in many countries, though not all), are at the forefront and in the middle of these complex sociocultural and political discourses that influence childbirth practices. Childbirth practices – the overall delivery of service provision and individual acts of care, procedures or interventions carried out by obstetricians and midwives – have significant ramifications on the experiences and life courses of those receiving care (Renfrew et al., 2014). Concurrently, how people experience and interpret receiving care and their birth experiences is also shaped by biopsychosocial-cultural expectations (Davis-Floyd & Cheyney, 2009; Downe et al., 2018). These are continually shaped and co-constructed within societies as tides turn, favour shifts, wants or expectations change. Birth can be a highly contested and politically charged space, with vehement views often in opposition[1]. For some, physiological birth and midwifery care is the anathema to quality maternity care. For others, me included, both physiological birth (where this is safe and possible[2]) and midwifery care are viewed as having intrinsic value. Although, these are not mutually exclusive, as some women will birth uneventfully without a midwife (McKenzie & Montgomery, 2021). Moreover, quality, skilled, relational midwifery care supersedes the eventual mode of birth (Tunçalp et al., 2015; White Ribbon Alliance, 2013; WHO, 2021). Where midwifery care is grounded in respectful and dignified care, the overall biopsychosocial experience and outcomes are enhanced regardless of whether a birth was physiological or required medical support or intervention (Morton & Simkin, 2019; Shakibazadeh et al., 2018).[3] Therefore, midwifery care is vital for all women during birth. These views are supported by robust international evidence explored in this chapter and the next.

Midwifery as a profession, midwives as individuals, face ongoing power battles within the professional space of caregiving – often positioned as subservient to obstetric practices and institutional demands (McFarland et al., 2019).[4] Moreover, internationally, midwifery and midwives are undervalued with marked underinvestment – demonstrated by the growing global crisis of workforce shortages (UNFPA et al., 2021). Lack of investment in a neoliberal capitalist society indicates where power holders (those with political and financial power) perceive value (Dahlen, H. et al., 2022; Fine & Saad-Filho, 2017). Low investment in midwifery and midwives indicates low status and value, mirroring the broader undervaluing of women, childbearing and mothering (Filby et al., 2016; Renfrew & Malata, 2021). With quality midwifery demonstrating positive benefits for over 56 maternal and neonatal outcomes including reductions in maternal mortality and infant stillbirths (Renfrew et al., 2014), lack of investment and valuing of midwifery has serious consequences (Kennedy et al., 2018; Renfrew & Malata, 2021). The burden of underinvestment and poor outcomes are mostly felt by low-income countries (Filby et al., 2016), where 'too little medicine' such as resources, facilities, life-saving medications or interventions and skilled care is patchy, entirely lacking or inaccessible to women (Miller et al., 2016). However, issues within high-income countries are typically felt to be around 'too much medicine' (Miller et al., 2016) where the overuse of medical interventions tips over from beneficial to becoming harmful (WHO, 2018b). While this is a crude simplification, the issues are more complex; essentially, there is a global midwifery and birthing crisis (White Ribbon Alliance, 2022). While unevenly distributed, even in places with midwives as lead professionals for childbearing women, struggles with underinvestment, inadequate pay and working conditions have created dangerous shortages (UNFPA et al., 2021);[5] and power struggles continue (White Ribbon Alliance, 2022). Crucially, these issues (and many more) detrimentally impact childbearing outcomes: physically, mentally and emotionally with far-reaching consequences across the mother-baby dyad's life courses.

'Normal' physiological birth is also a contested site with associated power struggles (Lyerly, 2012; Lynch, 2020; Royal College of Midwives, 2022c). The use of the word 'normal' and its direct implications in comparison to what is deemed 'abnormal', over time, has been critiqued around implicit or explicit moralising or stigmatising judgements (Bartlett, 2011; Rost, 2021; Winance, 2007). However, in terms of 'normal birth', this term has typically been used as an abridged colloquialism referring to 'normal physiological labour and birth' – the biological processes of labour and birth which have been studied through the basic sciences, anatomy, physiology, epidemiology, observational and interventional studies. This body of evidence is not a moral judgment of 'normal vs abnormal' to which critics claim (Lyerly, 2012); rather, through these studies, the parameters of a physiological birth have been broadly determined, international definitions generated and complications of birth studied to help identify key markers for births that require lifesaving assistance (Renfrew et al., 2014; WHO, 2018a). Broadly, physiological birth is one where labour starts spontaneously, proceeds without incident (problem or emergency), nor requires intervention, and results in a spontaneous birth, with mother and baby well.[6] The conflation of normal physiological birth with 'any' vaginal birth that may involve induction, augmentation and instrumental birth has added heat to a polarised debate (Beech, 2017; Feeley, 2021). Moreover, there are concerns that proponents of (exclusively) medicalised births are against the *concept* of normal physiological labour and birth rather than the language of 'normal' (Beech, 2017; Gutteridge, 2022), to which compelling arguments exist (outlined above). Those against the concept of physiological labour and birth contradict the compelling international qualitative insights finding that most women (not all) anticipate and want a normal physiological birth, crucially, expecting their maternity caregiver to be skilled to facilitate that safely (Downe et al., 2018).[7]

A 'normal' physiological birth has important psychosocial and biological benefits for mothers and babies (Renfrew & Malata, 2021; The Lancet, 2018). Physiological births are associated with enhanced experiences of a positive birth (Hildingsoon et al., 2013; Olza et al., 2018), greater levels of maternal-infant attachment (Romano & Lothian, 2008), less infant complications such as respiratory or other chronic metabolic illnesses (Dahlen, H. et al., 2013), (including less respiratory disorders in children up to 16 years old) (Dahlen, H. et al., 2021), higher breastfeeding initiation and continuation rates which have significant maternal-infant health benefits (Rollins et al., 2016), and reduced complications in subsequent pregnancies (WHO, 2018c). The benefits of physiological births are also related to reducing the potential harms of *routine*[8] interventions including induction of labour, augmentation of labour, continuous electronic monitoring, episiotomies, instrumental births, or caesarean sections (ten Hoope-Bender et al., 2014; The Lancet, 2018). These routine procedures are often associated with hospital institutionalised birth practices (Johanson et al., 2002). Although many procedures can be lifesaving (The Lancet, 2018), the exponential rise in birth interventions over the past 20–30 years have raised concerns that too much medicine outweighs the benefits of their use, thus causing iatrogenic harm (Renfrew et al., 2014; WHO, 2018c). Recent international efforts have focused attention on reducing unnecessary and harmful interventions signalling a shift away from unwarranted medical technocratic birth practices.[9]

Getting the balance of 'enough medicine' (and/or care), not too much, not too little, is an essential component of quality maternity care (Miller et al., 2016). To which, midwifery is vital both to ensure the protection of physiological processes and to provide timely appropriate referrals or lifesaving interventions (Renfrew et al., 2014). The Lancet Midwifery Series (Renfrew et al., 2014), the largest review carried out, examined 13 meta-syntheses and 173 systematic reviews that determined that midwifery 'is a vital solution to the challenges of providing high-quality maternal and newborn care for all women and newborn infants, in all countries' (p. 8). Moreover, central to quality midwifery/maternity[10] care is the relational aspects between the mother-caregiver (Walsh & Devane, 2012). When meaningful relationships are cultivated, trust and mutual respect occur, women's experiences are enhanced, and safety within a holistic perspective is ensured (Downe et al., 2018; Walsh & Devane, 2012).[11] The bedrock of relational care is centring on the needs of birthing women and people, working in partnership and collaboration, and affirming their human rights and dignity throughout (Shakibazadeh et al., 2018). This includes supporting autonomous decision-making, irrespective of the beliefs held by the midwife or obstetrician. Facilitating or ensuring women's agency is a core component of midwifery practice, underpinned by respectful care, an enabling relationship ensures power and control remain held by the woman with positive benefits beyond the birth experience (Thomson & Feeley, 2019). Where women feel disempowered, disrespected, or experience a lack of control, evidence demonstrates a long-lasting negative impact, including birth trauma (Reed et al., 2017).

'Alternative' physiological birth: Autonomy, choice and tensions

Having defined and explained physiological birth, in this research, I defined 'alternative' physiological birth choices as 'birth choices that go outside of local/national maternity guidelines or when women decline recommended treatment of care, in the pursuit of a physiological birth' (Feeley, 2019). Such characterisation excludes birth choices that go outside of maternity guidelines where women are seeking increased medical surveillance and/or medical interventions such as elective induction of labour or caesarean. The distinction between both types of birth choices is important. The premise for this research relates to dominant sociocultural-political discourses of medicalisation, technocratic, risk-averse and institutionalisation that has shaped childbirth practices in the UK (and beyond).[12] These discourses have been attributed to creating hegemonic birth practices (Clesse et al., 2018) to the detriment of physiological birth rates (WHO, 2018c), women's choices when seeking a physiological birth (Holten & de Miranda, 2016) and midwives' ability to provide evidence-based and woman-centred care within their skillset of facilitating physiological birth (Cooper, 2011; Davis & Homer, 2016; Newnham & Kirkham, 2019). This focus does not negate the importance of supporting *all* birth choices and women's autonomy – which is central to ethical care. However, physiological birth and 'alternative physiological birth' fall under the direct remit of midwifery practice, as mentioned, a site for tensions and conflict that this research sought to explore. Moreover, within the context of declining physiological birth rates, exploring 'alternative' physiological births provides a window to examine the sociocultural-political complexities around birth practices, autonomy, choice, and their tensions.

The ability/opportunity for women to make 'choices' during pregnancy and childbirth is embedded within governmental policies, cultural norms and women's expectations. Such rhetoric is also associated with the global movement for improved human rights during childbirth that includes respect for women's decision-making and autonomy, including the right to decline recommended care or treatment (ICI, 2021; White Ribbon Alliance, 2011). However, evidence suggests that women can face opposition, conflict, reprisals and restrictive care provision when they attempt to challenge technocratic, medicalised, risk-averse and institutionalised hegemonic birth practices (Feeley & Thomson, 2016a; Roberts & Walsh, 2018).[13] Alternative physiological birth choices, as previously defined, may include healthy women declining routine maternity care practices such as labour induction after 41 weeks of gestation, or vaginal examinations to assess the progress of labour or fetal monitoring during labour. Other situations include women who have had medical or obstetric risk factors seeking midwifery-led care and/or non-obstetric settings (home or birth centres). Decisions that resist these discourses can be perceived as controversial despite legislation that assures women's bodily autonomy and rights to choose their care.

Although studies have explored women's decision-making and experiences of alternative physiological birthing choices[14], few at the time of this research had examined the views and experiences of midwives caring for them.[15] This was an important gap as 'full-scope' midwifery as defined by the Lancet (Renfrew et al., 2014), includes the optimisation of normal biological, psychological, social and cultural processes whilst respecting women's individual circumstances and views. Therefore, the facilitation of alternative physiological births directly falls within this remit and concurs with the international definition of midwifery (International Confederation of Midwives, 2014, 2017) and the midwifery philosophy of woman-centred individualised care (Bradfield et al., 2018). This lack of attention was and still is significant because women's ability to assert their agency can be influenced positively or negatively by their midwife caregivers (Coxon et al., 2017). Such influence may be related to the midwives' personal philosophy of childbirth (Cooper, 2011), personal experiences of birth (Church, 2014), professional experiences of birth (Daemers et al., 2017), skill sets (Walker et al., 2018), perceptions of risk (Coxon et al., 2017) or how they value women's autonomy (Kruske et al., 2013).

In addition, midwives' ability to practice can be influenced positively or negatively by their sociocultural and political working contexts (Newnham & Kirkham, 2019; Nilsson et al., 2019), with of course additional challenges now related to the COVID-19 pandemic (Berg et al., 2022). In the UK, and other similar high-income contexts most women receive care commissioned by institutions (e.g., the UK NHS). Although institutions such as the NHS have excellent outcomes at the population level (DH, 2021),[16] its scale lends itself to routine, procedural, bureaucratic-driven care at the expense of individualised, relational care, women's ability to assert agency and their experiences of care (further discussed in Chapter 2). Moreover, organisational issues such as medicalised, risk-averse, technocratic cultures, poor staffing and busy workloads can limit midwives' ability to practice autonomously (Davis & Homer, 2016; Vermeulen et al., 2019). As such, institutional limitations to midwifery practice can adversely affect women's access to individualised woman-centred care and skilled physiological birth care. For example, evidence shows for similar cohorts of women (health status/risk profile), *where* they give birth strongly influences their outcomes i.e., significantly less likelihood of a physiological birth in hospital settings (Brocklehurst, 2011; Reitsma et al., 2020).[17] It is within findings such as these that we can explore the institutional and sociocultural-political impact and influence upon birth practices and outcomes.

A core issue within institutional maternity care can be captured as 'guideline-centred' care (Kotaska, 2011). Guidelines are used throughout health and social care in the UK (also common elsewhere) and are embedded into governance processes, procedures and insurance statuses of hospitals (Weisz et al., 2007). Used well, guidelines are structured documents with focused information about a given topic including care practice information on what to consider doing, when and why. Used poorly, guidelines distil and perpetuate routine, procedural and bureaucratic-driven care at the expense of individual patient autonomy and professional expertise (Greenhalgh, 2018; Wieringa & Greenhalgh, 2015). Issues arise when they are used as 'rule books' – a prescriptive approach to healthcare whereby punitive action may occur should a professional or a person receiving care does not follow the prescribed guideline (Alexander & Bogossian, 2018; Symon, 2000). As an unintended consequence of the proliferation of guidelines across healthcare, alongside astounding maternity litigation claims, guideline adherence has become synonymous with 'safe' care or rather, care that can be defended in the event of a claim (Alexander & Bogossian, 2018; Griffith & Tengnah, 2010). Therefore, opting 'outside of guidelines', the basis of this study, can be viewed as deviant or problematic, *despite* the centrality of individualised care within policy, legislation, international and national guidance and professional obligations[18] to ensure care wraps around the needs of those receiving care. The chasm between policy rhetoric, legislation, best practice and the reality for both professionals and birthing women is central to this research whereby significant tensions between large-scale institutional delivery of maternity services, individualised care and physiological birth exist.

Independent and employed midwives

It is important to differentiate between independent/private and employed midwives. Central to this book are the experiences of employed midwives delivering alternative physiological birth care within the constraints of institutional working. While the place of midwifery practice may be different (community, birth centre or hospital), employed midwives are subjected to employee obligations, expectations and terms of their contract. Some employee requirements are explicit and failing to adhere would mean termination of the contract (Royal College of Midwives, 2022a). Other requirements are implicit, cultural artefacts such as strict guideline adherence are subject to interpretation depending on the organisational, social and political culture (Feeley et al., 2021). While there are enormous challenges for midwives working independently (self-employed) across the globe, they do have relative autonomy and freedom to practice without rigid structures associated with large-scale organisational working. Broadly, independent midwives are known for providing a 'gold standard of care' – a case-loading model in which they are the sole care provider for a particular woman and family throughout the childbearing journey (Frohlich, 2007). This way of working allows the time and space to build intimate trusting relationships without the bureaucratic and time pressures employed midwives face (Wickham, 2010). By virtue of this way of working, individualised care irrespective of health status can be actualised. Therefore, independent midwives are well known for their skills and desire to support alternative physiological births. This was captured in a systematic review (Feeley et al., 2019) of the literature that explored midwives' views of these birthing decisions and found independent midwives 'willingly facilitative' of these birth choices – based on strongly held beliefs of women's autonomy coupled with appropriate skills to deliver this care.

However, independent midwifery practice is also subjected to ongoing political battles. For example, in the UK, independent midwives had been denied insurance products since June 2020 (IMUK, 2020), which has only recently been resolved (Zest, 2022).[19] In the US, midwives in some states are not recognised legally and professionally; thus, integration into the wider health system is inconsistent (Vedam et al., 2018). New Zealand has had an established model of independent midwives (Lead Maternity Care Providers) reimbursed by the government to deliver care (Grigg & Tracy, 2013). However, low pay and poor working conditions have stimulated several court proceedings to address pay inequity and discrimination (New Zealand College of Midwives, 2017). Echoing New Zealand, Canadian midwives working within a similar model of independence renumerated by the government, have won three court proceedings regarding poor inequitable pay, yet the government is yet to provide the pay lift they have been awarded (Association of Ontario Midwives, 2022). Drawing attention to the challenges independent midwives face further highlights the impact of broader sociocultural-political issues already discussed. Given the world is short of 900,000 midwives (UNFPA et al., 2021), the issues independent midwives face reiterate the overall undervaluing of the profession and the benefits to a childbearing population. While the rest of this book focuses on employed midwives, it is important to recognise independent midwifery is also a site for political struggle and tension, albeit with different challenges to those employed.

The research

This book centres on research that captured narrative accounts and interviews from NHS-employed midwives, who were self-defined as facilitative of alternative physiological birth choices. The research was underpinned by a feminist pragmatist theoretical framework that ontologically focuses on 'real world' problems whereby knowledge generation is utilised to affect positive social change (Fischer, 2014; Seigfried, 1996). Feminist pragmatists are aligned with pragmatist perspectives in conjunction with broad feminist theories that perceive that knowledge is constructed, contingent and intrinsically political (McHugh, 2015). Therefore, feminist pragmatism inherently adopts a critical perspective to account for issues of gender, power and structural influences in people's experiences, the meaning-making attributed to experiences as well as the production of knowledge (Fischer, 2014; Seigfried, 1996). Feminist pragmatism was justified for this study as the research questions pose a feminist inquiry – it centers on midwives' (a female-dominated profession) and women's birth choices. Women's bodies as a site for power, control and regulation have long been discussed (Davis-Floyd & Cheyney, 2009; Kitzinger, 2005; Newnham, 2014), with feminists arguing that structural paternalism marginalises women's ways of knowing, access to equitable services and autonomous decision making. Additionally, the midwifery profession is also a site for power, control and regulation as outlined in this chapter. In this study, midwives were viewed as 'situated knowers' (McHugh, 2015) with the capacity to generate bottom-up, practice-based knowledge. By using a narrative research methodology, where stories/narratives are viewed as knowledge devices (Bamberg, 2010), the midwives' situated knowledge was captured and analysed via stories of professional practice.

45 midwives generously gave up their time to participate, to share their practice-based stories and experiences of delivering this type of maternity care. My

core focus was to collect practice-based stories that related to any physiological birth choice deemed outside of the guidelines. Taking such a broad approach was to move beyond specific decisions or clinical scenarios such as focusing only on home vaginal birth after caesarean or water breech births etc. Instead, the aim was to develop practice-based knowledge and insights that could be applied to any birth choice, to elucidate the principles of midwifery practice in this context as well as examine the experiences and sociocultural-political influences on delivering 'out of guidelines' care. Accordingly, I had three key research questions to answer, to find out how midwives delivered this care so that practice-based evidence could be used for other midwives and maternity professionals within their practice. I also wanted to understand their experiences of doing so, what was it like for the midwives? Then taking a broader view, I wanted to examine the intersection, influence and impact of social, cultural and political discourses on their practice and experiences in delivering care. To answer these three research questions, three different narrative analyses were carried out, one building on the other.[20]

The midwives recruited for the study were mostly employed by different organisations (known as hospital Trusts)[21] from across the UK. This provided data and analyses to generate broader insights and perspectives, beyond that of a localised culture, for the same reason as above. The midwife participants were diverse in several ways (see Appendix 1): working in different settings (community, birth centres, hospital), working in different roles, in different models (continuity or fragmented), with different levels of experience (<2 years qualified to >30) and levels of seniority (junior/senior/management). Such diversity strengthened the findings, moving the discussion beyond specific midwifery settings, models and levels of experience, demonstrating this type of care is not contingent on particular parameters which may be subject to polarisation i.e. home vs hospital, continuity vs fragmented models of care, inexperienced vs experienced midwives, junior/seniority, etc. This study demonstrates that facilitating alternative physiological births is within the remit of any and all midwives across all maternity settings.

I invited the midwives to either write a reflective account (self-written narrative) or have an interview, with many opting to do both. Starting with an open question, the midwives either wrote or told me about a specific alternative physiological birth they had facilitated. In interviews, this initial practice example paved the way for a wide-ranging conversation that spanned numerous alternative physiological births, the midwives' own experiences of birth, their attitudes and beliefs etc. In all the interviews and some of the written accounts, the midwives wove in stories about their workplace environments and how where they worked affected them personally, through the caregiving approach they adopted. Some were heart breaking accounts of isolation, ostracisation and bullying. Others were uplifting accounts of workplace friendship, camaraderie and support. All, of course, worked within the same broad societal landscape of opposing and conflicting sociocultural-political discourses, so for their experiences to be so different was a surprising element of the study.

It is also important to note the context at the time of recruitment. Data was collected in 2017, during a time of great change, the Francis (2013) and Kirkup (2015) reports exposed two failing hospitals with significant implications for maternity services. Among many changes, this resulted in supervision[22] being removed from legislative statute (DH, 2017; Parliamentary and Health Service Ombudsman, 2013), Nursing and Midwifery Council[23] changes (DH, 2017; NMC, 2015), increased scrutiny and concerns around 'normal' birth including a turn in media reporting condemning midwives, midwifery practice and 'normal' birth (Darling, 2021; Spain, 2022). More recently, the publication of the Ockendon Report (2022) exposed maternity service failings within another Trust, to which midwives and physiological birth have come under greater pressure by the media.[24] These challenges, further contextualised by 12 years of austerity, Brexit and the COVID-19 pandemic have co-created significant workforce issues around recruitment, retention and appropriately skilled maternity provision (Royal College of Midwives, 2022b). Thus, the UK landscape for the midwife participants was rocky then and has been increasingly destabilised since. Particularly around the value of midwifery care, women's choices and physiological birth practices – homebirth, birth centre and waterbirth services are frequently closed, continuity teams are being disbanded (Birthrights, 2022), and greater paternalistic narratives dominate the UK landscape. Therefore, the study findings maintain relevance and are perhaps needed more now than before. As polarised debates deepen in the UK, we must learn from midwives who are practising within the system to support birthing women and people's physiological birth choices.

Conclusion

This chapter has set the scene for this book and the research carried out. While the findings presented have been collected from a UK context, they resonate across different high-income country contexts. For example, researchers in the Netherlands, Australia, the US and Canada have been asking similar questions, exploring the nature of maternity service provision and whether it meets women's needs (or not) – see endnote 14. Moreover, having presented at many international conferences and webinars, the feedback from many international midwives is one of resonance with their working context. However, international differences exist in terms of what may be deemed 'alternative' or out of guidelines. For example, Newnham et al. (2018) situate homebirth itself as an alternative birth choice and water birth in Hong Kong may be deemed alternative.[25] Notwithstanding these specific differences, again highlighting the influence of sociocultural-political contexts, the core message remains – women's choices for physiological birth and midwives' ability to deliver the care women want and expect are frequently constrained. 'Not being allowed' to do the job they are educated to do is a recurring message of why midwives leave the profession (RCM, 2016; UNFPA et al., 2021; White Ribbon Alliance, 2022). While what midwives (and women) are not allowed to do may look different in different countries, and some of the examples presented in this book may feel extraordinarily radical to some midwives, the broad issues are persistently consistent. In the next chapter, we will explore the intersecting discourses that give rise to hegemonic birth practices to create tensions between the rhetoric and reality of supporting and facilitating physiological birth.

Notes

1 For example, homebirth is a contested space internationally. A meta-analysis carried out by Wax et al. (2010) cited an alarming tripling of neonatal mortality. This generated a significant number of refutations, example here (Sandall et al., 2011) and the Editor's of AJOG responding to the number of letters they received (AJOG Editorial Team, 2011). This is one example of many areas of contention across the physiological birth with longstanding discussion and disagreements generally framed as a dichotomy as either 'birth as a risky event', only safe in retrospect or 'birth as a normal life event' sometimes requiring help/interventions (Johanson et al., 2002). While the conversation is moving on to consider humanised birth approaches, appropriate and judicious interventions for the right person at the right time, see Miller et al. (2016), dichotomous thinking is still evident in practice. As the birth binaries has been the subject of many books and articles, I have refrained from too much detail here, assuming you, the reader is aware of these issues.

2 Being physiologically informed does not negate the necessity for appropriate, judicious medical interventions where that is needed and wanted by birthing women and people (Feeley et al., 2020).

3 The converse is also true with growing evidence indicating that 'birth trauma' may be reconceptualised as 'maternity care trauma' as studies find negative, disrespectful, undignified care and fractured relationships with maternity providers as a leading cause of distress and traumatic experience see- (Bohren et al., 2015; Feeley & Thomson, 2016b; Reed et al., 2017; Thomson & Downe, 2008).

4 Longstanding power struggles have been analysed and critiqued by several feminist academics. In brief, midwives have been demonised since the Middle Ages (Newnham, 2014). Further vilification occurred during the 17th and 18th century, as centuries of systematic exclusion of women from medicine, science and religion entered the birthing sphere (Cahill, 2000). Stacey (1988) suggested that the small number of men-midwives that began to successfully deliver (live) babies with forceps challenged the tradition of birth within the female domestic arena. Capitalising upon the emergence of 'scientific knowledge' as morally superior, a systematic devaluing of midwifery 'traditional' knowledge occurred (Cahill, 2000; Stacey, 1988). The rise of the medical market, medical 'professionalisation' and subsequent dominance of doctors grew in all areas of health whereby to assert authority required a proactive strategy to vilify and undermine midwives (amongst other competitors) (Stacey, 1988).

5 This report was published in 2021, since then, growing news coverage from a range of countries report a 'mass exodus' of midwives and/or ongoing shortages. For example, Canada https://globalnews.ca/news/8813886/midwife-shortage-abbotsford-bc/; Australia https://www.theguardian.com/australia-news/2022/apr/13/babies-missing-out-on-health-checks-in-melbourne-due-to-covid-related-workforce-shortagestheUKhttps://inews.co.uk/news/health/top-midwife-maternity-shortage-increasingly-more-difficult-safe-care-1550717; New Zealand https://www.nzherald.co.nz/bay-of-plenty-times/news/bay-of-plenty-midwife-shortage-midwives-from-other-regions-called-to-help/2EBFSKFDH ETQXASLHO4LDVZR4A/#:~:text = While %20 the %20 Bay %20 of %20 Plenty, throughout %20 New %20 Zealand %20 Maternity %20 Services.

6 There are some variations across the globe regarding the definition of a physiological birth, often the 'risk' status of the woman will be used to define a normal physiological birth i.e. low risk at the onset of labour (and remaining low risk) and/or where the fetus is head down rather than breech presenting (International Confederation, 2014; WHO, 1996), to which there is some disagreement. For example, those with obstetric or medical complexities often will go into spontaneous labour, proceed without complication or intervention and have a spontaneous physiological birth – such is the subject of this study! Therefore, I've opted to use this broad definition to circumvent these debatable variations.

7 The qualitative systematic review while finding that most women desired and anticipated a normal birth, women were also prepared that labour and/or birth may require assistance or intervention, recognising there was need to 'go with the flow' (Downe et al., 2018), therefore, women's expectations around a normal birth are not 'at any cost'.

8 These interventions can be lifesaving, however, the balance tips to harm when used routinely, injudiciously.

9 See (Miller et al., 2016; Renfrew & Malata, 2021; Renfrew et al., 2014; ten Hoope-Bender et al., 2014; The Lancet, 2018; WHO, 2018c).

10 Relational care characterised by meaningful connection and trust is essential for all health and social care professionals. However, in maternity care, its presence or absence has an exceptionally strong impact due to the emotional and life-long impact of childbearing.

11 Concepts of safety in maternity care will be explored further in Chapter 2, however, it is essential to view safety within a broader lens and must include psychological, cultural and spiritual safety.

12 For an insightful and recent global perspective, see the special issue in Health, Risk & Society. It includes sophisticated considerations of these issues, collating papers from Brazil, Jordan, Switzerland, Turkey, China, Japan, Italy and Senegal (Topçu & Brown, 2019).

13 Also see (Jackson et al., 2012; Keedle et al., 2015; Plested & Kirkham, 2016; Scamell, 2014; Shallow, 2013; Viisainen, 2000) to name a few studies.

14 Studies have explored women's experiences of alternative birth choices include: freebirthing, which is an active decision to give birth with no professional's present (Dahlen, H. G. et al., 2011; Feeley & Thomson, 2016; Freeze & Tanner, 2020; Jackson et al., 2012; McKenzie & Montgomery, 2021; Miller, A. C., 2009); 'high-risk' homebirths (Hollander, Holten, Leusink et al., 2018); vaginal birth after caesarean (VBAC) at home or in a birth pool (Keedle et al., 2015; McKenna & Symon, 2014).

15 Exploring the experiences of maternity professionals in relation to alternative physiological births is now a rapidly growing area of international scholarship e.g. the Netherlands (Hollander et al., 2019), Canada (Wines, 2016), Australia (Jenkinson et al., 2017). While the book Birthing outside the system: The canary in the coalmine largely focused on women's motivations and experiences, several chapters share insights from maternity professionals (Dahlen, H. et al., 2020). Additionally, with personal contact with many researchers in this field, new studies are in their early stages of development.

16 Although, to caveat this point, significant disparities exist in high-income countries – Black, Asian and women from minority groups experience worse maternal/neonatal outcomes, with Black women suffering the most significant impact (Adane et al., 2020; Howell, 2018; Knight et al., 2022; Urquia et al., 2017).

17 The findings from the UK Birthplace Study (Brocklehurst, 2011) demonstrated the relationship between the intended place of birth with birth outcomes in 64,538 low risk women. It found that women (of similar cohorts, health and risk status) were significantly less likely to have a vaginal birth if they planned to birth in an OU i.e. 58%, compared to; 76% for planned births at a birth centre attached to hospital, 83% for

planned births at a free-standing birth centre, 88% for planned births at home. These are collated figures of both first and second (or more) time mothers. These figures demonstrate that for the majority of (low risk) women choosing to birth in hospital reduces their chance of a physiological birth and its associated benefits.

18 In the UK, (similar to many countries) health professionals are regulated. Their regulators set down frameworks of expected practice health professionals are duty bound to follow. Personalised, individualised care is a common professional obligation, yet, is found lacking due to institutional constraints such as an over emphasis on complying with guidelines.

19 Lack of political will to address the UK Independent Midwives (IM) insurance is ongoing – despite the profound impact that COVID-19 has had on NHS midwives and women's choices such as homebirth service suspensions, to which IM's could have been enabled to provide (IMUK, 2020). (This was true at the time of writing, however, now a product has been found (Zest, 2022), but only due to tenacious midwives making it happen.)

20 I have purposefully avoided including dense methodological information, hoping to ensure this book is accessible to all readers. For those interested in extensive methodological insights please see (Feeley, 2019).

21 In the UK, the NHS is divided into 'hospital Trusts' which are commissioned to deliver services in specific geographical areas. A 'Trust' providing maternity services typically includes hospital settings (the dominant place), community midwifery services for homebirth provision, antenatal/postnatal care (sometimes in conjunction with GP surgeries) and may include birth centre provision (free standing or adjoined within the hospital). Therefore, a 'Trust' is responsible for all maternity service provision, employment of the staff across the different areas, and operate under the same employment contracts, policies, guidelines etc.

22 For midwifery, supervision was a statutory responsibility which provided a mechanism for support and guidance to every midwife practising in the UK. The stated purpose of supervision of midwives was to protect women and babies by actively promoting a safe standard of midwifery practice, however, failings of this mechanism were found in the Francis Report which led to its statutory removal (Francis, 2013; Parliamentary and Health Service Ombudsman, 2013).

23 The NMC is the regulatory body for nurses and midwives in the UK and were implicated in the failings at Morecombe Bay (Francis, 2013; Parliamentary and Health Service Ombudsman, 2013).

24 Media reporting of the Ockendon report has focused onerously on midwifery care and physiological birth, despite tragic outcomes being evidenced as 'routine medicalised approaches to birth' such as high levels of induction, syntocinon, poorly skilled obstetric instrumental births which coupled along with poor staffing and teamwork arguably, co-created poor outcomes, rather than physiological labour and birth per se. The conflation between 'any' vaginal birth and physiological birth as defined here has been a source of much tension and debate see my analysis (Feeley, 2021). Moreover, the Ockendon Report highlighted managerial cover-ups, poor governance structures and processes for investigations when adverse events occurred – these components are beyond the remit of most midwives and obstetricians in everyday practice (Ockendon, 2022).

25 During my MSc I had the pleasure of learning with 20+ midwives from Hong Kong who joined us at the University of Central Lancashire for a 'normal' birth module. During this intensive week they shared their clinical practice and working contexts which included their limitations, such as water for labour/birth is not typically facilitated. I was unable to find academic references to this point, but have included reports to illustrate this example of what is deemed 'alternative' differs depending on the context, see http://tyr.jour.hkbu.edu.hk/2013/03/20/water-birth-yet-to-gain-acceptance/ https://www.otandp.com/blog/water-birth-in-hong-kong

References

Adane, A. A., Farrant, B. M., Marriott, R., White, S. W., Bailey, H. D., & Shepherd, C. C. J. (2020). Socioethnic disparities in severe maternal morbidity in Western Australia: A statewide retrospective cohort study. *BMJ Open*, 10(11), e039260. doi: 10.1136/bmjopen-2020-039260

AJOG Editorial Team. (2011). Editors' comment. *American Journal of Obstetrics & Gynecology*, 204(4), e20. doi: 10.1016/j.ajog.2011.01.041

Alexander, C. R., & Bogossian, F. (2018). Midwives and clinical investigation: A review of the literature. *Women and Birth: Journal of the Australian College of Midwives*, 31(6), 442–452. doi: 10.1016/j.wombi.2018.02.003

Association of Ontario Midwives. (2022). Closing the gap: Understanding Ontario midwives' legal action. Association of Ontario Midwives. https://www.ontariomidwives.ca/closing-gap-understanding-ontario-midwives-legal-action

Bamberg, M. (Ed.). (2010). *Narrative Analysis*. APA Press, Washington

Bartlett, S. (2011). *Normality Does Not Equal Mental Health: The Need to Look Elsewhere for Standards of Good Psychological Health*. Praeger/ABC-CLIO.

Beech, B. (2017). *The backlash against Normal Birth*. AIMS.org.uk. https://www.aims.org.uk/campaigning/item/the-backlash-against-normal-birth

Berg, L. v. d., Thomson, G., Jonge, A. d., Balaam, M., Moncrieff, G., Topalidou, A., & Downe, S. (2022). 'Never waste a crisis': A commentary on the COVID-19 pandemic as a driver for innovation in maternity care. *BJOG: An International Journal of Obstetrics & Gynaecology*, 129(1), 3–8. doi: 10.1111/1471-0528.16996

Birthrights. (2022). *Coronavirus*. birthrights.org.uk. https://www.birthrights.org.uk/campaigns-research/coronavirus/

Bohren, M. A., Vogel, J. P., Hunter, E. C., Lutsiv, O., Makh, S. K., Souza, J. P., Aguiar, C., Saraiva Coneglian, F., Diniz, A. L. A., Tunçalp, Ö., Javadi, D., Oladapo, O. T., Khosla, R., Hindin, M. J., & Gülmezoglu, A. M. (2015). The mistreatment of women during childbirth in health facilities globally: A mixed-methods systematic review. *PLoS Medicine*, 12(6), e1001847; discussion e1001847. doi: 10.1371/journal.pmed.1001847

Bradfield, Z., Duggan, R., Hauck, Y., & Kelly, M. (2018). Midwives being 'with woman': An integrative review. *Women Birth*, 31(2), 143–152. doi: 10.1016/j.wombi.2017.07.011

Brocklehurst, P. (2011). Perinatal and maternal outcomes by planned place of birth for healthy women with low risk pregnancies: The Birthplace in England national prospective cohort study. *BMJ*, 343, d7400. doi: 10.1136/bmj.d7400

Cahill, H. (2000). Male appropriation and medicalization of childbirth: An historical analysis. *Journal of Advanced Nursing*, 33(3), 334–342.

Church, S. (2014). Midwives' personal experiences of pregnancy and childbirth: Exploring issues of autonomy and agency in relation to the use of professional knowledge. *Human Fertility* (Camb), 17(3), 231–235. doi: 10.3109/14647273.2014.949879

Clesse, C., Lighezzolo-Alnot, J., de Lavergne, S., Hamlin, S., & Scheffler, M. (2018). The evolution of birth medicalisation: A systematic review. *Midwifery*, 66, 161–167. doi: 10.1016/j.midw.2018.08.003

Cooper, T. (2011). *Perceptions of the Midwife's Role: A Feminist Technoscience Perspective*. University of Central Lancashire.

Coxon, K., Chisholm, A., Malouf, R., Rowe, R., & Hollowell, J. (2017). What influences birthplace preferences, choices and decision-making amongst healthy women with straightforward pregnancies in the UK? A qualitative evidence synthesis using a 'best fit' framework approach. *BMC Pregnancy and Childbirth*, 17(1). doi: 10.1186/s12884-017-1279-7

Daemers, D., van Limbeek, E., Wijnen, H., Nieuwenhuijze, M., & de Vries, R. (2017). Factors influencing the clinical decision-making of midwives: A qualitative study. *BMC Pregnancy and Childbirth*, 17(1). doi: 10.1186/s12884-017-1511-5

Dahlen, H., Drandic, D., Shah, N., Cadee, F., & Malata, A. (2022). Supporting midwifery is the answer to the wicked problems in maternity care. *The Lancet Global Health*, 10(7), e951–e952. doi: 10.1016/S2214-109X(22)00183-8

Dahlen, H., Jackson, M., & Stevens, J. (2011). Homebirth, freebirth and doulas: Casualty and consequences of a broken maternity system. *Women and Birth: Journal of the Australian College of Midwives*, 24(1), 47–50. doi: 10.1016/j.wombi.2010.11.002

Dahlen, H., Kennedy, H., Anderson, C., Bell, A., Clark, A., Foureur, M., Ohm, J., Shearman, A., Taylor, J., Wright, M., & Downe, S. (2013). The EPIIC hypothesis: Intrapartum effects on the neonatal epigenome and consequent health outcomes. *Medical Hypotheses*, 80(5), 656–662. doi: 10.1016/j.mehy.2013.01.017

Dahlen, H., Kumar-Hazard, B., & Schmied, V. (2020). *Birthing Outside the System: The Canary in the Coal Mine* (1st ed.). Routledge, Abingdon, Oxon.

Dahlen, H., Thornton, C., Downe, S., de Jonge, A., Seijmonsbergen-Schermers, A., Tracy, S., Tracy, M., Bisits, A., & Peters, L. (2021). Intrapartum interventions and outcomes for women and children following induction of labour at term in uncomplicated pregnancies: A 16-year population-based linked data study. *BMJ Open*, 11(6), e047040. doi: 10.1136/bmjopen-2020–047040

Darling, F. (2021). *"Normal birth at any cost" – Understanding and addressing root causes is important to promoting safety in UK maternity services.* https://www.all4maternity.com/normal-birth-at-any-cost-understanding-and-addressing-root-causes-is-important-to-promote-safety-in-uk-maternity-services/#:~:text=Introduction,only%20midwives%2C%20but%20also%20obstetricians

Davis, D., & Homer, C. S. E. (2016). Birthplace as the midwife's workplace: How does place of birth impact on midwives? *Women and Birth*, 29(5), 407–415. doi: 10.1016/j.wombi.2016.02.004

Davis-Floyd, R., & Cheyney, M. (2009). Birth and the big bad wolf: An evolutionary perspective. In H. Selin & P. Stone (Eds.), *Childbirth across Cultures: Ideas and Practices of Pregnancy, Childbirth, and the Postpartum* (pp. 1–22). Springer.

DH. (2017). *The Nursing and Midwifery Council – Amendments to Modernise Midwifery Regulation and Improve the Effectiveness and Efficiency of Fitness to Practise Processes Consultation Report.* Leeds: Department of Health. https://assets.publishing.service.gov.uk/government/uploads/system/uploads/attachment_data/file/582494/Consultation_report.pdf

DH. (2021). *Safer maternity care progress report 2021.* London: gov.uk. https://www.england.nhs.uk/wp-content/uploads/2021/03/agenda-item-9.4-safer-maternity-care-progress-report-2021-amended.pdf

Downe, S., Finlayson, K., Oladapo, O., Bonet, M., & Gülmezoglu, A. (2018). What matters to women during childbirth: A systematic qualitative review. 13(4). doi: 10.1371/journal.pone.0194906

Feeley, C. (2019). 'Practising outside of the box, whilst within the system': A feminist narrative inquiry of NHS midwives supporting and facilitating women's alternative physiological birthing choices. Doctoral Thesis: University of Central Lancashire. http://clok.uclan.ac.uk/30680/

Feeley, C. (2021). Normal birth – the scapegoat for poor maternity care. *Midwifery Matters*, (171), 16–19. https://www.midwifery.org.uk/articles/midwifery-matters-winter-2021-issue-171/

Feeley, C., Byrom, A., Byrom, S., & Tizard, H. (2020). Normal birth position statement. *The Practising Midwife*, 23(1), 34.

Feeley, C., & Thomson, G. (2016a). Tensions and conflicts in 'choice': Women's' experiences of freebirthing in the UK. *Midwifery*, 41, 16–21. doi: 10.1016/j.midw.2016.07.014

Feeley, C., & Thomson, G. (2016b). Why do some women choose to freebirth in the UK? An interpretative phenomenological study. *BMC Pregnancy and Childbirth*, 16, 59. doi: 10.1186/s12884-016-0847-6

Feeley, C., Thomson, G., & Downe, S. (2019). Caring for women making unconventional birth choices: A meta-ethnography exploring the views, attitudes, and experiences of midwives. *Midwifery*, 72, 50–59. doi: 10.1016/j.midw.2019.02.009

Filby, A., McConville, F., & Portela, A. (2016). What prevents quality midwifery care? A systematic mapping of barriers in low and middle income countries from the provider perspective. *Plos One*, 11(5). doi: 10.1371/journal.pone.0153391

Fine, B., & Saad-Filho, A. (2017). Thirteen things you need to know about neoliberalism. *Critical Sociology*, 43(4–5), 685–706. doi: 10.1177/0896920516655387

Fischer, C. (2014). *Gendered Readings of Change: A Feminist-Pragmatist Approach*. Palgrave Macmillan.

Francis, R. (2013). *Report of the Mid Staffordshire NHS Foundation Trust Public Inquiry Executive summary*. The Stationery Office Limited. https://assets.publishing.service.gov.uk/government/uploads/system/uploads/attachment_data/file/279124/0947.pdf

Freeze, R., & Tanner, L. (2020). Freebirth in the United States. In H. Dahlen, B. Kumar-Hazard & V. Schmied (Eds.), *Birthing Outside the System The Canary in the Coal Mine* (pp. 1–27). Routledge: Abingdon, Oxon.

Frohlich, J. (2007). Independent midwifery: A model of care on the brink of extinction. *MIDIRS Midwifery Digest*, 17(38), 213–218.

Greenhalgh, T. (2018). Of lamp posts, keys, and fabled drunkards: A perspectival tale of 4 guidelines. *Journal of Evaluation in Clinical Practice*, 24(5), 1132–1138. doi: 10.1111/jep.12925

Griffith, R., & Tengnah, C. (2010). *Law and Professional Issues in Midwifery (Transforming Midwifery Practice Series)*. Learning Matters Ltd, Exeter.

Grigg, C., & Tracy, S. (2013). New Zealand's unique maternity system. *Women and Birth: Journal of the Australian College of Midwives*, 26(1), 59. doi: 10.1016/j.wombi.2012.09.006

Gutteridge, K. (2022). *Silence is Never Golden-Midwives and women speaking out*. https://www.maternityandmidwifery.co.uk/silence-is-never-golden-midwives-and-women-speaking-out/

Hildingsoon, I., Johansson, M., KarlstrÃm, A., & Fenwick, J. (2013). Factors associated with a positive birth experience: An exploration of Swedish women's experiences. International Journal of Childbirth, 3(3), 153–164. doi: 10.1891/2156-5287.3.3.153

Hollander, M., Holten, L., Leusin, A., & van Dillen, J. (2018). Less or more? Maternal requests that go against medical advice. *Women & Birth*, 31(6), 505–512. doi: 10.1016/j.wombi.2018.01.010

Hollander, M., Holten, L., Leusink, A., van Dillen, J., & de Miranda, E. (2018). Less or more? Maternal requests that go against medical advice. *Women & Birth*, 31(6), 505–512. doi: 10.1016/j.wombi.2018.01.010

Hollander, M., Miranda, E., Vandenbussche, F., Dillen, J., & Holten, L. (2019). Addressing a need. Holistic midwifery in the Netherlands: A qualitative analysis. *Plos One*, 14(7). doi: 10.1371/journal.pone.0220489

Holten, L., & de Miranda, E. (2016). Women's motivations for having unassisted childbirth or high-risk homebirth: An exploration of the literature on 'birthing outside the system'. *Midwifery*, 38, 55–62. doi: 10.1016/j.midw.2016.03.010

Howell, E. (2018). Reducing disparities in severe maternal morbidity and mortality. *Clinical Obstetrics and Gynecology*, 61(2), 387–399. doi: 10.1097/GRF.0000000000000349

ICI. (2021). *The International Childbirth Initiative (ICI) the 12 steps (summary version) to safe and respectful motherbaby-family maternity care.* https://icichildbirth.org/wp-content/uploads/2021/05/ICI_12StepSummary2021.pdf

ICM. (2014). *Core document philosophy and model of midwifery care.* The Hague: ICM. https://www.internationalmidwives.org/assets/files/definitions-files/2018/06/eng-philosophy-and-model-of-midwifery-care.pdf

IMUK. (2020). *Statement on the Withdrawal of Professional Indemnity Insurance.* IMUK. https://imuk.org.uk/news/statement-on-the-withdrawal-of-professional-indemnity-insurance/

International Confederation of Midwives. (2017). *ICM Definitions: Definition of the Midwife.* https://www.internationalmidwives.org/our-work/policy-and-practice/icm-definitions.html

Jackson, M., Dahlen, H., & Schmied, V. (2012). Birthing outside the system: Perceptions of risk amongst Australian women who have freebirths and high-risk homebirths. *Midwifery*, 28(5), 561–567. doi: 10.1016/j.midw.2011.11.002

Jenkinson, B., Kruske, S., & Kildea, S. (2017). The experiences of women, midwives and obstetricians when women decline recommended maternity care: A feminist thematic analysis. *Midwifery*, 52. doi: 10.1016/j.midw.2017.05.006

Johanson, R., Newburn, M., & Macfarlane, A. (2002). Has the medicalisation of childbirth gone too far? *Bmj*, 324(7342), 892–895. doi: 10.1136/bmj.324.7342.892

Keedle, H., Schmied, V., Burns, E., & Dahlen, H. G. (2015). Women's reasons for, and experiences of, choosing a homebirth following a caesarean section. *BMC Pregnancy and Childbirth*, 15(1), 206. doi: 10.1186/s12884-015-0639-4

Kennedy, H. P., Cheyney, M., Dahlen, H. G., Downe, S., Foureur, M. J., Homer, C. S. E., Jefford, E., McFadden, A., Michel-Schuldt, M., Sandall, J., Soltani, H., Speciale, A. M., Stevens, J., Vedam, S., & Renfrew, M. J. (2018). Asking different questions: A call to action for research to improve the quality of care for every woman, every child. *Birth*, 45(3), 222–231. doi: 10.1111/birt.12361

Kirkup, B. (2015). *The Report of the Morecambe Bay Investigation. Morecambe Bay Investigation.* https://assets.publishing.service.gov.uk/government/uploads/system/uploads/attachment_data/file/408480/47487_MBI_Accessible_v0.1.pdf

Kitzinger, S. (2005). *The Politics of Birth.* Elsevier: Abingdon, Oxon.

Knight, M., Bunch, K., Vousden, N., Banerjee, A., Cox, P., Cross-Sudworth, F., Dhanjal, M. K., Douglas, J., Girling, J., Kenyon, S., Kotnis, R., Patel, R., Shakespeare, J., Tuffnell, D., Wilkinson, M., & Kurinczuk, J. J. (2022). A national cohort study and confidential enquiry to investigate ethnic disparities in maternal mortality. *eClinicalMedicine*, 43, 101237. doi: 10.1016/j.eclinm.2021.101237

Kotaska, A. (2011). Guideline-centered care: A two-edged sword. *Birth*, 38(2), 97–98.

Kruske, S., Young, K., Jenkinson, B., & Catchlove, A. (2013). Maternity care providers' perceptions of women's autonomy and the law. *BMC Pregnancy and Childbirth*, 13(1), 84. doi: 10.1186/1471-2393-13-84

Lyerly, A. (2012). Ethics and 'normal birth'. *Birth: Issues in Perinatal Care*, 39(4), 315–317.

Lynch, E. (2020). Normal birth: Contention and debate in the UK. *The Practising Midwife*, 23(8). https://www.all4maternity.com/normal-birth-contention-and-debate-in-the-uk/

McFarland, A. K., Jones, J., Luchsinger, J., Kissler, K., & Smith, D. C. (2019). The experiences of midwives in integrated maternity care: A qualitative metasynthesis. *Midwifery*, 80, 102544. doi: 10.1016/j.midw.2019.102544

McHugh, N. (2015). *The Limits of Knowledge: Generating Pragmatist Feminist Cases for Situated Knowing.* State University of New York Press, New York.

McKenna, J. A., & Symon, A. G. (2014). Water VBAC: Exploring a new frontier for women's autonomy. *Midwifery*, 30(1), e20–e25. doi: 10.1016/j.midw.2013.10.004

McKenzie, G., & Montgomery, E. (2021). Undisturbed physiological birth: Insights from women who freebirth in the United Kingdom. *Midwifery*, 101, 103042. doi: 10.1016/j.midw.2021.103042

Miller, A. C. (2009). "Midwife to myself": Birth narratives among women choosing unassisted homebirth★. *Sociological Inquiry*, 79(1), 51–74. doi: 10.1111/j.1475-682X.2008.00272.x

Miller, Abalos, E., Chamillard, M., Ciapponi, A., Colaci, D., Comandé, D., Diaz, V., Geller, S., Hanson, C., Langer, A., Manuelli, V., Millar, K., Morhason-Bello, I., Castro, C., Pileggi, V., Robinson, N., Skaer, M., Souza, J., Vogel, J., & Althabe, F. (2016). Beyond too little, too late and too much, too soon: A pathway towards evidence-based, respectful maternity care worldwide. *Lancet*, 388(10056), 2176–2192. doi: 10.1016/S0140-6736(16)31472-6

Morton, C., & Simkin, P. (2019). Can respectful maternity care save and improve lives? Birth, 46(3), 391–395. doi: 10.1111/birt.12444

New Zealand College of Midwives. (2017). *Historic win for midwives.* Midwifery News. https://www.midwife.org.nz/wp-content/uploads/2019/02/Pages-from-Midwifery-News-85-June-2017-hi-res.pdf

Newnham, E. (2014). Birth control: Power/knowledge in the politics of birth. *Health Sociology Review*, 23(3), 254–268. doi: 10.1080/14461242.2014.11081978

Newnham, E., & Kirkham, M. (2019). Beyond autonomy: Care ethics for midwifery and the humanization of birth. *Nursing Ethics*, 26(7–8), 2147–2157. doi: 10.1177/0969733018819119

Newnham, E., McKellar, L., & Pincombe, J. (2018). Introduction. In E. Newnham, L. McKellar & J. Pincombe (Eds.), *Towards the Humanisation of Birth: A Study of Epidural Analgesia and Hospital Birth Culture* (pp. 1–15). Palgrave Macmillan.

Nilsson, C., Olafsdottir, O. A., Lundgren, I., Berg, M., & Dellenborg, L. (2019). Midwives' care on a labour ward prior to the introduction of a midwifery model of care: A field of tension. *International Journal of Qualitative Studies on Health and Well-Being*, 14(1). doi: 10.1080/17482631.2019.1593037

NMC. (2015). Francis Report: Position statement. nmc.org.uk. https://www.nmc.org.uk/about-us/policy/position-statements/francis-report/#:~:text=Robert%20Francis'%20thorough%20report%20outlines, learnt%20from%20the%20Francis%20report

Ockendon, D. (2022). *Findings, conclusions and essential actions from the independent review of maternity services at the Shrewsbury and Telford Hospital NHS Trust.* London: HH Associates Ltd. https://www.gov.uk/government/publications/final-report-of-the-ockenden-review

Olza, I., Leahy-Warren, P., Benyamini, Y., Kazmierczak, M., Karlsdottir, S., Spyridou, A., Crespo-Mirasol, E., TakÃ¡cs, L., Hall, P., Murphy, M., Jonsdottir, S., Downe, S., & Nieuwenhuijze, M. (2018). Women's psychological experiences of physiological childbirth: a meta-synthesis. *BMJ Open*, 8(10). doi: 10.1136/bmjopen-2017–020347

Parliamentary and Health Service Ombudsman. (2013). *Midwifery supervision and regulation: Recommendations for change.* The Stationery Office Limited. https://www.ombudsman.org.uk/

Plested, M., & Kirkham, M. (2016). Risk and fear in the lived experience of birth without a midwife. *Midwifery*, 38, 29–34. doi: 10.1016/j.midw.2016.02.009

RCM. (2016). *Why midwives leave revisited.* London: RCM. https://www.proquest.com/openview/914f52ff00a17d34da28f892b2d4985d/1.pdf?pq-origsite=gscholar&cbl=506295

Reed, R., Sharman, R., & Inglis, C. (2017). Women's descriptions of childbirth trauma relating to care provider actions and interactions. *BMC Pregnancy and Childbirth*, 17. doi: 10.1186/s12884-016-1197-0

Reitsma, A., Simioni, J., Brunton, G., Kaufman, K., & Hutton, E. K. (2020). Maternal outcomes and birth interventions among women who begin labour intending to give birth at home compared to women of low obstetrical risk who intend to give birth in hospital: A systematic review and meta-analyses. *The Lancet*, 21(100319), e100319.

Renfrew, M., McFadden, A., Bastos, M., Campbell, J., Channon, A., Cheung, N., Silva, D., Downe, S., Kennedy, H., Malata, A., McCormick, F., Wick, L., & Declercq, E. (2014). Midwifery and quality care: Findings from a new evidence-informed framework for maternal and newborn care. *Lancet*, 384(9948), 1129–1145. doi: 10.1016/S0140-6736(14)60789-3

Renfrew, M., & Malata, A. (2021). Scaling up care by midwives must now be a global priority. *The Lancet Global Health*, 9(1), e2–e3. doi: 10.1016/S2214-109X(20)30478-2

Roberts, J., & Walsh, D. (2018). Babies come when they are ready: Women's experiences of resisting the medicalisation of prolonged pregnancy. *Feminism & Psychology*, 29(1), 40–57. doi: 10.1177/0959353518799386

Rollins, N., Bhandari, N., Hajeebhoy, N., Horton, S., Lutter, C., Martines, J., Piwoz, E., Richter, L., & Victora, C. (2016). Why invest, and what it will take to improve breastfeeding practices? *The Lancet*, 387(10017), 491–504. https://doi.org/10.1016/S0140-6736(15)01044-2

Romano, A., & Lothian, J. (2008). Promoting, protecting, and supporting normal birth: A look at the evidence. *Journal of Obstetric, Gynecologic, and Neonatal Nursing: JOGNN/NAACOG*, 37(1), 94–105. doi: 10.1111/j.1552-6909.2007.00210.x

Rost, M. (2021). "To normalize is to impose a requirement on an existence." Why health professionals should think twice before using the term "normal" with patients. *Journal of Bioethical Inquiry*, 18(3), 389–394. doi: 10.1007/s11673-021-10122-2

Royal College of Midwives. (2022a). *Care outside guidance: Caring for those women seeking choices that fall outside guidance*. London: Royal College of Midwives. https://www.rcm.org.uk/media/5941/care_outside_guidance.pdf

Royal College of Midwives. (2022b). *Midwife numbers now lower than at the last general election says RCM*. rcm.org.uk. https://www.rcm.org.uk/media-releases/2022/march/midwife-numbers-now-lower-than-at-the-last-general-election-says-rcm/

Royal College of Midwives. (2022c). *Re:Birth Summary Report*. London: Royal College of Midwives. https://www.rcm.org.uk/media/6234/re_birth_summary_.pdf

Sandall, J., Bewley, S., & Newburn, M. (2011). "Home birth triples the neonatal death rate": Public communication of bad science? *American Journal of Obstetrics and Gynecology*, 204(4), e17–e18. doi: 10.1016/j.ajog.2011.01.036

Scamell, M. (2014). 'She can't come here!' Ethics and the case of birth centre admission policy in the UK. *Journal of Medical Ethics*, 40(12), 813–816.

Seigfried, C. (1996). *Pragmatism and Feminism: Reweaving the Social Fabric*. University of Chicago Press, Chicago.

Shakibazadeh, E., Namadian, M., Bohren, M. A., Vogel, J. P., Rashidian, A., Nogueira Pileggi, V., Madeira, S., Leathersich, S., Tunçalp, Ö, Oladapo, O. T., Souza, J. P., & Gülmezoglu, A. M. (2018). Respectful care during childbirth in health facilities globally: A qualitative evidence synthesis. *BJOG: An International Journal of Obstetrics and Gynaecology*, 125(8), 932–942. doi: 10.1111/1471–0528.15015

Shallow, H. (2013). Deviant mothers and midwives: supporting VBAC with women as real partners in decision making. *Essentially MIDIRS*, 4(1), 17–21.

Spain, H. (2022). This Hurts: how the media portrays childbirth matters. *Aims*, 34(2). https://www.aims.org.uk/journal/item/obstetric-violence-media?fbclid=IwAR 1eE5VfStQrtstT4Q2W_osL1RkAthlTgYpPskzjdgGuMecJFTH7lYNDMoM

Stacey, M. (1988). *The Sociology of Health and Healing*. Unwin Hyman, London.

Symon, A. (2000). Litigation and defensive clinical practice: Quantifying the problem. *Midwifery*, 16(1), 8–14. doi: 10.1054/midw.1999.0181

ten Hoope-Bender, P., de Bernis, L., Campbell, J., Downe, S., Fauveau, V., Fogstad, H., Homer, C., Kennedy, H., Matthews, Z., McFadden, A., Renfrew, M., & Van Lerberghe, W. (2014). Improvement of maternal and newborn health through midwifery. *Lancet*, 384(9949), 1226–1235. doi: 10.1016/S0140-6736(14)60930-2

The Lancet. (2018). Stemming the global caesarean section epidemic. *Lancet*, 392(10155). doi: 10.1016/S0140-6736(18)32394-8

Thomson, G., & Downe, S. (2008). Widening the trauma discourse: The link between childbirth and experiences of abuse. *Journal of Psychosomatic Obstetrics & Gynaecology*, 29(4), 268–273.

Thomson, G., & Feeley, C. (2019). The 'trusting communion' of a positive birth: An existential perspective. In S. Downe, & S. Byrom (Eds.), *Squaring the Circle: Normal Birth Research Theory And Practice In A Technological Age* (pp. 47–53). Pinter & Martin, London.

Topçu, S., & Brown, P. (2019). The impact of technology on pregnancy and childbirth: creating and managing obstetrical risk in different cultural and socio-economic contexts. *Health, Risk & Society*, 21(3–4), 89–99. doi: 10.1080/13698575.2019.1649922

Tunçalp, Ö, Were, W. M., MacLennan, C., Oladapo, O. T., Gülmezoglu, A. M., Bahl, R., Daelmans, B., Mathai, M., Say, L., Kristensen, F., Temmerman, M., & Bustreo, F. (2015). Quality of care for pregnant women and newborns—the WHO vision. *Bjog*, 122(8), 1045–1049. doi: 10.1111/1471-0528.13451

UNFPA, ICM, & WHO. (2021). *The state of the world's midwifery: 2021*. UNFPA. https://www.unfpa.org/sowmy

Urquia, M. L., Wanigaratne, S., Ray, J. G., & Joseph, K. S. (2017). Severe maternal morbidity associated with maternal birthplace: A population-based register study. *Journal of Obstetrics and Gynaecology Canada*, 39(11), 978–987. doi: 10.1016/j.jogc.2017.05.012

Vedam, S., Stoll, K., MacDorman, M., Declercq, E., Cramer, R., Cheyney, M., Fisher, T., Butt, E., Yang, Y. T., & Powell Kennedy, H. (2018). Mapping integration of midwives across the United States: Impact on access, equity, and outcomes. *PLoS One*, 13(2). 10.1371/journal.pone.0192523

Vermeulen, J., Luyben, A., O'Connell, R., Gillen, P., Escuriet, R., & Fleming, V. (2019). Failure or progress?: The current state of the professionalisation of midwifery in Europe. *European Journal of Midwifery*, 3(December), 22. 10.18332/ejm/115038

Viisainen, K. (2000). The moral dangers of home birth: Parents' perceptions of risks in home birth in Finland. *Sociology of Health & Illness*, 22(6), 792–814. doi: 10.1111/1467-9566.00231

Walker, S., Batinelli, L., Rocca-Ihenacho, L., & McCourt, C. (2018). 'Keeping birth normal': Exploratory evaluation of a training package for midwives in an inner-city, alongside midwifery unit. *Midwifery*, 60, 1–8. doi: 10.1016/j.midw.2018.01.011

Walsh, D., & Devane, D. (2012). A metasynthesis of midwife-led care. *Qualitative Health Research*, 22(7), 897–910.

Wax, J. R., Lucas, F. L., Lamont, M., Pinette, M. G., Cartin, A., & Blackstone, J. (2010). Maternal and newborn outcomes in planned home birth vs planned hospital births: A metaanalysis. *American Journal of Obstetrics and Gynecology*, 203(3), 243.e1–243.e8. doi: 10.1016/j.ajog.2010.05.028

Weisz, G., Cambrosio, A., Keating, P., Knaapen, L., Schlich, T., & Tournay, V. (2007). The emergence of clinical practice guidelines. *The Milbank Quarterly*, 85(4), 691–727. doi: 10.1111/j.1468-0009.2007.00505.x

White Ribbon Alliance. (2011). *Respectful maternity care: The universal rights of childbearing women*. Washington: White Ribbon Alliance.

White Ribbon Alliance. (2013). *5 approaches to respectful maternity care*. https://www.ohchr.org/sites/default/files/Documents/Issues/Women/SR/Reproductive HealthCare/White_Ribbon_Alliance.docx

White Ribbon Alliance. (2022). What women want: Midwives' voices, midwives' demands. Washington, DC: WRA. https://www.whiteribbonalliance.org/wp-content/uploads/2022/05/MidwivesVoicesMidwivesDemands_GlobalReport.pdf?eType=EmailBlastContent&eId=a911eecc-5149-463d-8c5c-7e7bab8aeea4

WHO. (1996). *Care in Normal Birth: A Practical Guide*. Geneva: World Health Organization.

WHO. (2018a). *WHO Recommendations Intrapartum Care for a Positive Childbirth Experience*. Geneva: World Health Organisation.

WHO. (2018b). *WHO Recommendations Non-Clinical Interventions to Reduce Unnecessary Caesarean Sections*. Geneva: World Health Organisation. http://apps.who.int/iris/bitstream/handle/10665/275377/9789241550338-eng.pdf?ua=1

WHO. (2018c). *WHO recommendations non-clinical interventions to reduce unnecessary caesarean sections*. Geneva: World Health Organization. https://apps.who.int/iris/bitstream/handle/10665/275377/9789241550338-eng.pdf

WHO. (2021). *WHO Recommendation on Effective Communication between Maternity Care Providers and Women in Labour*. Geneva, Switzerland: WHO. https://srhr.org/rhl/article/who-recommendation-on-effective-communication-between-maternity-care-providers-and-women-in-labour

Wickham, S. (2010). Journeying with women: Holistic midwives and relationships. *Birthspirit Midwifery Journal*, 6, 15–21.

Wieringa, S., & Greenhalgh, T. (2015). 10 years of mindlines: A systematic review and commentary. *Implementation Science*, 10(45), 1–11.

Winance, M. (2007). Being normally different? Changes to normalization processes: From alignment to work on the norm. *Disability & Society*, 22(6), 625–638. doi: 10.1080/09687590701560261

Wines, J. (2016). Could the midwives of British Columbia benefit from a model of midwifery supervision? Master's Thesis: University of Central Lancashire. (Available on request)

Zest (2022). Midwifery in the UK is changing. Available at https://www.zestmidwives.co.uk/. Retrieved 27th November 2022

2

RHETORIC VS. REALITY

The power of hegemonic birth practices

Chapter 1 positioned physiological labour and birth as having value with health and wellbeing benefits for the mother-baby dyad across their life-courses, and established that quality midwifery care is a means to facilitate physiological labour and birth safely. Drawing upon international perspectives, we explored some of the tensions that arise generally around physiological birth and midwifery care, thus paving the way to consider the premise of this research – physiological birth choices 'outside of guidelines.' Such choices may be considered deviant, with evidence demonstrating that birthing women and people face challenges and obstacles when asserting their agency. This chapter will provide a closer examination of these challenges, providing the context for the study. First, an examination of UK maternity services will be presented. As a site for tensions and contradictions, I will highlight that the reality for service users does not always match the rhetoric. Second, to understand these tensions, key sociocultural-political influences will be explored, which I will argue to coalesce as 'guideline-centred' care. Guideline-centred care is the crux of this research, for, without this, the concept of women 'going outside' of guidelines would not be problematic; for it is within this space, obstacles arise for both women and caregivers.

Rhetoric vs. reality

The UK maternity context is a conflicted space. Despite a strong professional midwifery workforce to deliver both personalised care and provide safe physiological labour and birth care, such birth rates are at an all-time low (NMPA, 2019). Despite strong evidence, policy and infrastructure (access to emergency obstetric or paediatric care) in support of all four birth places (home, adjoining maternity units, freestanding maternity units and obstetric units); births in midwifery-led settings and subsequent physiological birth rates remain low

DOI: 10.4324/9781003265443-2

(NHS Digital, 2021; Walsh et al., 2018). The UK has strong national policy and guidelines in favour of individualised or personalised care (NHS England, 2016; NHS England and Improvement, 2021), with robust legislation to support maternal autonomy (RC M, 2022). Yet evidence suggests service-users experience otherwise, particularly those seeking non-standardised care (Birthrights, 2022a; Roberts & Walsh, 2018). Accordingly, there is a significant disparity between maternity care rhetoric and the current reality. While the COVID-19 pandemic has placed a huge strain on maternity services and professionals and has compounded pre-existing problems (Berg, L. et al., 2022; Brigante et al., 2022), the issues explored below, predate the pandemic.

As stated, the UK has a strong professional midwifery workforce embedded within an integrated maternity system across all birth settings (home, birth centres and hospital), with timely access to medical or paediatric care, should the need arise. International evidence demonstrates midwifery-led care and midwifery-led settings are associated with fewer interventions and complications, more spontaneous vaginal birth rates and positive experiences of care (Hodnett et al., 2012; Reitsma et al., 2020; Sandall et al., 2016). Therefore, the UK maternity system should, in theory, generate high rates of safe, physiologically normal births,[1] and positive experiences. However, a decline in physiological birth rates has been observed over the past 30 years (Kennedy et al., 2018). For example, in England, NHS Digital (2018) showed in 2017–2018, spontaneous onset of labour was at a low rate of 52% (compared to 68% ten years previously), spontaneous birth at 58% (compared to 62% ten years previously), induction rates were 32% (compared to 20% ten years previously), and caesarean section rates were 28% (compared to 25% ten years previously). The most recent data from 2020–2021 demonstrated further decline – the spontaneous onset of labour was 47% and spontaneous birth was 53% (NHS Digital, 2021). Furthermore, these statistics hide several routine interventions such as artificial rupture of membranes, augmentation with syntocinon and episiotomies (Birth Choice, 2015; Dodwell, 2012; Downe & Finlayson, 2016). Therefore, rates of physiological labour and birth, as defined in Chapter 1 (page 3) are likely lower than reported. Other countries, such as the Nordic countries and the Netherlands, fare far better, without compromising maternal or neonatal wellbeing (Euro-Peristat Project, 2018). Reasons for the decline in physiological labour and births are multifaceted and complex – explored later in this chapter.

Within this context, for those wanting and anticipating a physiological birth, international research has demonstrated women expect their caregivers to be skilled to facilitate this competently and safely (Downe et al., 2018), arguably an appropriate expectation of maternity professionals. However, evidence shows for planned hospital births, similar cohorts of women (healthy, low risk of complications) are less likely to labour without interventions than those planning to birth in community settings (Brocklehurst, 2011; Burns et al., 2012). Therefore, raising concerns about the hospital environment, where most women give birth, is less conducive for those expecting physiological labour and birth care

(Goldkuhl et al., 2022). Moreover, a lack of exposure to physiological birth may negatively influence the skill acquisition and competencies of maternity professionals (McCourt et al., 2016; Russell, 2011), further compounding issues of lower physiological birth rates within hospital settings. Where community birthplace (home/FMU) settings are strongly associated with greater levels of physiological births, and fewer interventions and complications,[2] they often lack resource prioritisation to maintain the services (Beech, 2016; Walsh et al., 2018),[3] magnifying issues of exposure, skill acquisition and exacerbating the decline in physiological birth. Such issues are compounded by systemic issues, discussed below, limiting birthing women and people's access to enabling environments (health systems, services and providers) for competent physiological birth care. This contradicts the aim of UK policies which have centred on individualised, woman and person-centred care since 1993 (DH, 1993; DH, 2007; DH, 2010; England, 2017; NHS England, 2016). Now called 'personalised care' – asserting people should have choice and control and receive care based on what matters to them (NHS England, 2016; NHS England and Improvement, 2021).

Additionally, other difficulties exist for those seeking physiological birth care. While barriers can occur for women seeking access to more medical care such as elective caesareans or pharmacological pain relief (Birthrights, 2018; Thomson et al., 2019), evidence suggests for women making choices not culturally normative (i.e., in hospitals with routine medical interventions and/or with pharmacological pain relief) can experience moralistic opposition and restrictive care provision (Keedle et al., 2015; Shallow, 2013). These challenges occur despite robust legislation in support of maternal autonomy and agency, as described in Chapter 1. Examples of where physiological birth choice becomes compromised include limited access to homebirth services (Lee et al., 2016; RCM, 2011) and gatekeeping of birth centres (Scamell, 2014) or birth pools (Russell, 2011). Moreover, on the occasions when birthing women and people decline aspects of care – a core tenet of lawful informed consent – their ability to assert their agency may be compromised.[4] Newnham & Kirkham (2019) argue autonomy and informed consent are largely rhetorical within current maternity systems. For birthing women and people who do adhere to and agree with medical recommendations then autonomy may be perceived as being enabled. However, for those who disagree with such recommendations, opting for alternative approaches, and/or declining aspects of care, an unravelling of the commitments to autonomy and informed consent can occur through persuasion, coercion, threats and withdrawal of care (Newnham & Kirkham, 2019).

Coercive practices include repetitive discussions regarding the risks of the woman's decision (Plested & Kirkham, 2016), attempting to influence family members (Feeley & Thomson, 2016), threats or actual referrals to social services (McMahon & Ashworth, 2020), and the infamous 'dead baby' card – an articulation the baby might die if the woman does not comply with recommendations (Reed et al., 2017). Or less overtly, 'protective steering' may occur whereby conversations and information are controlled by health professionals either to protect women from perceived bad decision-making or to protect themselves as professionals (Levy, 1999). Self-protectionism may arise as maternity professionals have reported feeling pressure to conform to local guidelines and policies fearing disciplinary actions from their employers (Griffith & Tengnah, 2010; Robertson & Thomson, 2016). Thus, the tensions and contradictions existing within the UK maternity system expose the reality in stark contrast to the rhetoric. The next section explores the systemic issues that give rise to the challenges for those seeking midwifery-led care, midwifery-led birthplaces and/or physiological labour and birth, which can be largely attributed to 'hegemonic birth practices'.

Understanding the why: Sociocultural-political drivers

Having explored the contradictions existing within UK maternity services, this section examines key contributing factors to why choice and agency towards physiological birth, particularly those deemed 'alternative' can be problematic. Issues of medicalisation, institutionalisation, the misapplication of evidence-based medicine, constructs of safety, risk and litigation discourses align as hegemonic birth practices – negatively influencing physiological birth care, practices and experiences.[5] Moreover, medical hegemony has co-created a climate of fear and defensive practice, inhibiting authentic autonomous decision-making and caregiving which can be expressed as 'guideline-centred care' – a super-valuing of medical guidelines over personalised care approaches. Guideline-centred care is at the crux of this research, which is opposed to personalised, individualised care; the legal, moral and ethical framework to which maternity services should be delivered. That is not to say guidelines do not have a role in healthcare. Indeed, they do. However, used inappropriately and as an artefact of medical hegemony, their dominance exerts excessive authority and power over service users and maternity professionals alike. It is within this context, the notion of going 'outside of the guidelines' is laden with meaning, leading to the negative ramifications outlined in the previous section.

Medicalisation

Medicalisation has been defined as the process by which some aspects of human life, not previously considered pathological, come to be considered medical problems, leading to incumbent medical management (Maturo, 2012). As a social process, an expert-based biomedical paradigm dominates discussions, framing health/wellbeing in negative ways; defining or redefining illnesses and pathologies requiring medical treatment (Maturo, 2012). Critics argue the biomedical model of health offers a narrowed and limited focus on people's life courses marginalising the sociocultural context and individual meaning-making of what may be considered health or ill-health (Illich, 1975; Johanson et al., 2002; Maturo, 2012). Illich (1975) long raised concerns about 'the medicalisation of life' (p. 1). His argument centred around how the dominance of medicine and associated technologies were super-valued over environmental factors that contributed to ill-health such as food security, food quality, working conditions and sanitation (Illich, 1975). He argued social and political changes were required to make improvements to population health rather than medicine and biotechnology. Concerned about the 'medical enterprise' dominating normal human processes such as birth, death, and bereavement, Illich (1975) suggested it had caused unhealthy dependency, and reduced people's self-efficacy creating passive medical consumers which in turn has compounded medical dominance. A concern that continues to this day (Abbasi, 2022).

Related to childbirth, the biomedical model depicts a cultural shift from pregnancy and birth practised within a social sphere i.e., historically birth occurred at home with a female birth attendant or midwife, to one practised within a medical sphere i.e., birth mostly occurring in hospitals where medical management is directed by doctors (Newnham, E., 2014; van Teijlingen, 2005). The medical model is underpinned by a pathological approach to pregnancy and childbirth, whereby the major concern is to identify, reduce or treat 'risk' using surveillance, technology, and intervention; historically, related to the Cartesian mind-body dualism philosophical approach to medical practice and research (Wieringa, 2017). The body was the main concern of medicine, perceived as a 'machine' explained and understood by its individual parts (Haslem, 2011; Martin, 1987). Within childbirth, such a reductive perspective has been criticised by feminists that pregnancy and birth rendered women's bodies in mechanistic terms, an object to be 'done to' (van Teijlingen, 2005). Women's pregnant bodies became a site for power and control as male barber surgeons took an interest in childbearing women (Cahill, 2000; Stacey, 1988). The classic example of such practices was the development of the forceps by the Chamberlen family (Sheikh et al., 2013). This not only created a technology which opened access to male barber-surgeons to labouring women but, because the Chamberlen family did not allow midwives to use forceps, it also created a role division between competing birth attendant cadres (Sheikh et al., 2013).

Some researchers argue the biomedical model of birth was a professional project of subjugation, power and control by doctors over women's bodies/lives and encroached upon female midwives'/birth attendants' role in supporting childbirth (Cahill, 2000; Kitzinger, 2005; Oakley, 1986; Stacey, 1988). However, others suggest women were active agents in the cultural acceptability of the biomedical model, and it has brought many positive benefits such as lifesaving treatments and access to pharmacological pain relief (Beckett, 2005; Riessman, 1983). First-wave feminism is attributed to calls for access to pain relief and women were politically motivated to campaign for the right to relieve their suffering during childbirth (Beckett, 2005; Riessman, 1983). Beckett (2005) suggests this early activism created a mixed effect, success for the right to pain relief and obstetricians to consider pain relief methods. Yet women arguably facilitated the medicalisation process, losing control over childbirth including losing the comforts of home and support of female relatives and midwives.

Conversely, later, 'natural childbirth' movements are associated with second-wave feminism. This arose during the 1960s and 1970s as a response to medicalised, institutionalised, and technocratic births (Kitzinger, 2005). Within this model, resisting medicalisation occurred via seeking homebirths, the rise of birth plans, resisting paternalism, and resisting pharmacology by means of coping with birth. However, critics argued the natural birth movement was an essentialist paradigm, morally super-valuing 'natural' over medical care (Annandale & Clark, 1996; Beckett, 2005). Recent moves within the third wave of feminism support women's birthing choices of any kind (Beckett, 2005). Associated with neoliberal notions of individualism and choice (Thwaites, 2017), medicine or technology is not necessarily viewed as controlling and paternalistic, but rather viewed as offering emancipation from the pain of childbirth (Beckett, 2005).[6] However, critics argue that individualism and choice marginalise structural inequalities, and view the social construction of choice as politically constrained and often inequitable (Budgeon, 2015; McAra-Couper et al., 2011). Subsequently, in many cases, women's choices in childbirth are skewed towards medicalised approaches (Klein et al., 2006)[7] and in other cases, structural inequalities such as race, class and socioeconomic status may limit women's access to appropriate medical care (Birthrights, 2022b; Brubaker & Dillaway, 2009) with significant consequences such as higher mortality rates for Black women (MBRRACE-UK, 2021).

Overall disagreements regarding the positive and negative aspects of a medical approach to childbirth exist, with feminists on either side of the debate. An alternative view from Campbell and Porter (1997), who rather than accept dualities, conceptualised the feminist arguments as 'continua':

> … we would regard as ends of continua which stretch between the enablement and constraint of women's autonomy and the promotion and undermining of women's health … Our position contains value assumptions, namely that the enablement of autonomy is preferable to its constraint and the promotion of health is preferable to its undermining. Assuming acceptance of such values, the question then becomes one of deciding, on the basis of available evidence, toward which direction along the continua do specific modes of health care gravitate. (p. 356)

A systematic review regarding the medicalisation of birth supports this notion and situates it within a 'humanised birth' paradigm (Clesse et al., 2018). They suggest a humanised approach to birth can combine the positive effects of medicalisation whilst containing the iatrogenic harms. In this model, a physiological and holistic perspective of birth is held, women's needs are at the centre of care, and judicious use of medical interventions is applied, resisting routine approaches and the excesses of medicalisation (Clesse et al., 2018; Newnham, E. et al., 2018).

Therefore, the ideal scenario is that birthing women and people are enabled for their birth preferences in either direction (toward or away from a medicalised birth). However, the dominance of biomedicine (coupled with the discourses discussed below) frequently constrains choices for less medical intervention, as discussed in the previous section. As an illustration, a study by Roberts and Walsh (2018) explored women's experiences of resisting induction of labour for prolonged pregnancy and found women reported significant pressure to agree to an induction of labour to end the pregnancy. With medical induction, a normalised procedure/intervention, the women's decision to decline was frequently met with repetitive risk discussions and inference they were unduly putting their baby's life at risk by maternity professionals (Roberts & Walsh, 2018). Moreover, the pervasiveness of being 'overdue'- a medicalised construct, the women reported challenging social interactions with friends, family and even strangers offering unsolicited advice and challenging their decision to decline induction (Roberts & Walsh, 2018). This example echoes other situations where women decline aspects of care or seek midwifery-led models or birthplaces; not only do they experience pressure from health professionals to conform (Blaylock et al., 2022; Sanders & Crozier, 2018), but they also experience societal pressures (Naylor Smith et al., 2018; Skrondal et al., 2020). These situations challenge the idealised notion of third-wave feminism that all birthing choices are supported.

Institutionalised birth

In combination with a medicalised approach to birth, the shift from social birth spheres to medical spheres was associated with the rapid growth in hospital provision during the early 20th Century. For example, the expansion of medical jurisdiction over birth peaked with the shift to almost universal hospital births during the 1960s and 1970s in many high-income countries (Johanson et al., 2002; Newnham, 2014), with government policies reflecting and perpetuating the shift of birth to the hospital (Department, 1970; Newnham, 2014). Cahill (2000) and Newnham (2014) argue the hospital was pivotal to the rise of obstetric medicine (and arguably all medicine), a move not bound in evidence but based upon an assumption – access to doctors, medicine and technology was safer than the previous alternative (Cahill, 2000; Kitzinger, 2005; Newnham, 2014). However, Foucault (1973) asserted the rise of hospitals was not because they were safer or better, but as sites for information benefitting the growing medical profession. This coupled with wider societal changes influenced the cultural acceptance of hospitals as a safer place of birth (Behruzi et al., 2013). Therefore, a co-creation between women and maternity services has evolved – women's desires and needs are both constructed by and have constructed maternity care (De Vries, 1984), as highlighted earlier by the different waves of feminism. Therefore, rather than viewing women as victims of the sociocultural changes (though some were), women (mostly white middle class) have and continued to co-construct the sociocultural and political maternity landscapes (Behruzi et al., 2013). However, caution must be applied regarding *which* women's voices have catalysed these changes – for the negative consequences upon Black and Brown women are profound (Birthrights, 2022a) as are the devastating consequences of removing women from their Indigenous land to birth in hospitals (Cidro et al., 2020).

Moreover, concerns regarding the nature of institutions as big bureaucratic organisations where the needs of the institution are prioritised over the individual have been raised (Behruzi et al., 2013; Walsh, 2007). The nature of schedules and routine-based care can shape women's experiences of childbearing. For example, hospitals require schedules, which requires prioritising 'clock time' which runs counter to the natural rhythms of unpredictable labour (Martin, 1987; McCourt & Dykes, 2009). Therefore, routine medical management and interventions have been attributed to the need to manage the unpredictability of labour, and the 'smooth' running of hospital processes and procedures (Maher, 2008). Evidence has demonstrated that less physiological births occur within hospitals regardless of women's health status, highlighting the influence of place of birth (Brockle-hurst, 2011; Burns et al., 2012). Issues of task-based care, fragmented caregivers, and routine but potentially unnecessary interventions have been attributed to institutionalised birth practices (Kirkham, 2003; Walsh, 2006). Moreover, where UK Trusts delivers maternity services across community and hospital settings, hospitals tend to dominate resource allocation. Birth centres and homebirth services are likely to be suspended or closed in the event of staffing issues (Beech, 2016; Walsh et al., 2018), despite the evidence of their safety and efficacy. Centralisation of services reinforces the hospital as the default setting, reinforcing the medical model of birth. Therefore, there is an interdependent relationship between the medicalisation and institutionalisation of birth.

The emphasis on processes and procedures within hospitals has been said to mirror industrial production lines where efficiency is super-valued over individualised care delivery (Hunt & Symonds, 1995; Walsh, 2006). Within this model, fragmented care is the norm, and staff work shift patterns to suit the needs of the institution, thus not allowing for continuity of care (McCourt et al., 2011; Sheridan, 2010) nor cohesive inter-professional relationships (King's (Downe et al., 2010; Smith & Dixon, 2008). Such issues detrimentally affect the care women receive as well as the working cultural environment for midwives and their colleagues (NHS England, 2016). Poor intra and inter-professional working relationships have been related to poor outcomes for women and babies (King's Fund, 2012; Kirkup, 2015; Smith & Dixon, 2008). In addition, poor working relationships within hierarchal rigid institutionalised structures can manifest as a lack of trust among midwives, where toxic cultures of horizontal violence and bullying have been identified (Gillen et al., 2008; Leap, 1997). These issues are a contributing factor to midwives' dissatisfaction, high levels of stress and burnout and are leading reasons for midwives leaving the profession (Hunter et al., 2018).[8] In addition, women have reported a lack of dignified care, meaningful choices and poor birth experiences within institutionalised settings (Birthrights, 2013).

Standardisation is another sociocultural influence on birth practices associated with institutionalised healthcare. Standardisation promotes routinisation intending to improve efficiency and to a certain extent, to reduce variations in clinical practice and outcomes (Wears, 2015). Coupled with shifts toward quality improvement and governance structures, standardisation has become firmly embedded within maternity services, viewed as a mechanism for ensuring quality and accountability (Wears, 2015). For example, a standardised approach to antenatal care has been evidenced to benefit maternal-fetal health outcomes (WHO, 2016) and is offered to all women in the UK, thereby providing equitable care (NICE, 2021). However, standardised care does not work well in other maternity care situations and at times, contradicts individualised care (Reiger & Morton, 2012). For example, a standardised approach to the expected rate of cervical dilation during labour has resulted in many women being medically managed for 'failure to progress' (Abalos et al., 2018). A lack of attention to the 'unique normalness' of each woman's labour alongside hospital norms, routines and task-oriented care has meant standardised expectations can create iatrogenic harm (Downe & McCourt, 2004). Therefore, an uncritical adoption throughout maternity care has further entrenched medicalised-institutionalised birth practices (Downe, 2010; Reiger & Morton, 2012). Failing to account for complex systems, standardisation based upon a rationalist worldview seeks to simplify and control via methods of monitoring, evaluation and accountability (Wears, 2015). Such a reductive approach belies the 'reality of risk, ambiguity, chance and disorder' (Dekker & Nyce, 2012; Wears, 2015) – a site for challenge within maternity services. Moreover, it has created unwieldy scientific-bureaucratic systems which attempt to reduce complexities to simple procedures (Weisz et al., 2007). Excessive paperwork and a box-ticking approach have become commonplace, and bureaucratic-driven healthcare is the norm – taking time away from direct patient care that is in direct conflict with individualised caregiving, and a significant source of complaints (Reiger & Morton, 2012).

A product of standardisation, clinical guidelines, play a significant role within the sociocultural-political landscape of maternity services (and healthcare as a whole). Clinical guidelines are often understood as a product of evidence-based medicine (EBM). However, the production of guidelines predates notions of EBM (Weisz et al., 2007) and does not always correspond with the principles of EBM (Greenhalgh, 2014). Clinical practice guidelines are formalised documents which ideally combine the latest research, evaluated best medical evidence and expert consensus on the application of the research into a given area of clinical practice (Johannessen, 2017). Guidelines are used as a method of translating the evidence into usable documents for rapid dissemination to clinicians. They are used to standardise clinical practice and reduce clinical variations to improve the delivery of consistent, quality care to improve patient outcomes (Johannessen, 2017; Upshur, 2014). Guidelines are discretionary and require healthcare professionals to use their clinical expertise in applying them to provide the most appropriate care; any application of guidelines should be used in partnership with those receiving care, wherein their preferences must be *prioritised* and respected (Greenhalgh, 2015; Kotaska, 2011).

However, an over-reliance on guidelines has raised concerns,[9] particularly around creating a rule-based approach to healthcare, where deviations from the guidelines need to be justified (Downe, 2010; Griffith & Tengnah, 2010). Kotaska (2011) calls this 'guideline-centred care', which is in direct opposition to the woman-centred care approach espoused in UK maternity services. Downe (2010) suggested guidelines became de facto rules for health workers to follow, defendable in court should the situation arise. Conflation with employee policies and protocols that do require adherence[10] have further facilitated guidelines as 'rules' (McDonald et al., 2005); a dominating discourse whereby guideline adherence is prioritised over an individual's autonomy for fear of litigation and/or disciplinary action against the practitioner (Griffith & Tengnah, 2010; Ortashi et al., 2013). Medicalised, institutionalised, standardised (and governance) practices are distilled into guidelines (Arulkumaran, 2010). Guidelines, as an artefact of hegemonic birth practices, can be used to wield authority over women's access to types of care, for example, excluding women from birth centres if guidelines are operationalised on a 'rule-based' approach (Scamell, 2014). In these types of circumstances, guideline adherence becomes synonymous with 'safe' care, even where evidence exists to the contrary and contradicts the notion of personalised care.

Risk, governance, litigation and fearful defensive practice

The medicalisation and institutionalisation of birth have also been affected by other cultural shifts such as the safety/risk discourse. A 'risk society' borne from modernisation, the attempt of science to create order and control, has created a collection of *human-generated risks* requiring further control and management (Beck, 1992). Risk indicates the possibility of unintended and negative consequences of decisions or actions (Alaszewski et al., 1998). Therefore, risk management, particularly within healthcare, is concerned with regulating activities to reduce risks (Symon, 2000). Proliferating in the 1990s, multiple structures, organisational activities and mechanisms regarding performance, standardisation and accountability became embedded within healthcare; as such, organisational technologies have firmly entrenched a clinical governance culture and cultivated a 'risk aversion' lens to view healthcare services (Scamell, 2016). Furthermore, clinical governance does not appear to differentiate between 'human-generated risks' – iatrogenic harms and 'first order risk' – *potential* physiological hazards (Scamell, 2016). Iatrogenic harms include hospital-acquired infections, pressure ulcers and accidents – slips, trips and falls, and medication errors – as the responsibility of health services, risk management strategies are appropriate. In maternity care, prevention, detection and/or management of first-order risks such as pre-eclampsia or stillbirth are at the heart of quality maternity care (Scamell, 2016). However, applying risk management injudiciously to *potential* physiological hazards perpetuate overdiagnosis and overtreatments for the majority, unnecessarily creating iatrogenic harm (Rogers et al., 2019; Scamell, 2016).

Arguably, the risk and governance culture has conflated the management of institutional risk with physiological processes where 'safety' is reduced to and hyper-focused on physical outcomes during the childbearing continuum that can be controlled and managed (Healy et al., 2016; Scamell, 2016). However, this approach does not appear to recognise the iatrogenic harms caused by an over-reliance on a medicalised, interventionist approach to safety (Edwards et al., 2011; Kitzinger, 2005). For example, despite the known iatrogenic harms of several *routine* medical interventions or use of technology (i.e. continuous electronic fetal monitoring (CEFM) for healthy women including admission CEFM, augmentation of labour etc.) or those not demonstrating efficacy (four-hourly vaginal examinations, fetal blood sampling, prophylactic antibiotics in the absence of symptoms) (Renfrew et al., 2014) they continue to be used routinely (Downe & Finlayson, 2016).[11] The lack of implementation of known safe and beneficial practices (midwifery-led continuity of care, non-obstetric birthplaces, water immersion in labour etc.) (Renfrew et al., 2014) challenges the notions of a logical approach to risk management strategies. A further concern relates to the medicalisation of 'risk' – where the presence of risk factors for the disease has been elevated to the status of having the disease itself, which is then medically managed (Koerber et al., 2015).

Within these issues, attempting to discern what constitutes 'risk' or safety and from whose perspective is complex. With different and sometimes competing perspectives between intra and interprofessional groups, women and organisations/institutions, perceptions of risk are socially constructed and subjective. Subjectivity, individual perception, does not comfortably sit within a governance culture seeking to homogenise care and outcomes, or where there are perceived threats to organisational 'safety' e.g. its reputation,[12] therefore is a site of tension (Scamell, 2016). Such tensions relate to the 'labelling' of women as 'low' or 'high' risk which influences the care offered or withheld. Scamell & Alaszewski (2012) argued the political nature of maternity services and related risk discourses are represented by the narrowing parameters of normal birth. Healthy women at low risk of complications are provided care by midwives almost exclusively, therefore, professional tensions occur as definitions of risk evolve and change, and these boundaries are altered; women deemed at high risk often have limited choices such as place of birth, waterbirth or midwifery-led intrapartum care (Hunter & Segrott, 2014; Scamell & Alaszewski, 2012). In addition, the pervasiveness of the risk discourse has been found in midwives' accounts of fears even when supporting healthy women during the intrapartum period (Dahlen, 2010; Dahlen et al., 2014; Fenwick et al., 2012). Within this context, fears are likely to be heightened when women make decisions counter to medical or midwifery advice and/or organisational guidelines.

Issues of risk-averse discourses are bound in issues of blame, complaints, and litigation (Healy et al., 2016). Litigation is associated with the costs awarded to families if negligence has been proven to have caused a poor maternal or fetal outcome. Whilst data in the UK (2000–2009) demonstrated less than 0.1% of births have resulted in negligence claims, obstetric claims account for the largest awards paid to families (National Health Service, Litigation Authority, 2016).

More recently, of the total negligent claims paid out by the NHS in 2018–2019, £2.4bn, maternity accounted for 50%, raising significant concerns for the long-term sustainability of NHS healthcare provision (Yau et al., 2020). Complexities associated with the UK litigation system have stimulated an inadvertent 'blame' culture with distress and fear for families and professionals (Healy et al., 2016; Ortashi et al., 2013; Robertson & Thomson, 2016). The process of litigation has been historically slow,[13] contentious and highly stressful (Robertson & Thomson, 2016). Whilst current recommendations have suggested moves towards a no-blame compensatory award system in the event of adverse outcomes (NHS England, 2016), this is yet to be implemented in the UK. The benefits of such a system have been demonstrated in other countries and include an open and honest culture of learning when mistakes have been made, a non-punitive restorative approach to remedying clinician mistakes, improved safety and outcomes, and quicker financial compensation made available to the families to ensure their needs are met (NHS England, 2016).

Within 'blame' and litigious cultures, both midwives and doctors have reported cultures of fear and defensive practice (Alexander & Bogossian, 2018; Ortashi et al., 2013). Defensive practice has been defined as clinicians' deviation from their usual behaviour or good practice to reduce complaints, and criticism by either colleagues or families. However well-intentioned, defensive practice has been demonstrated to increase the use of (unnecessary) medicines, treatments, or interventions whilst clinicians err on the side of caution (Ortashi et al., 2013). Shorten (2010) refers to 'litigation-based practice' as opposed to evidence-based practice, suggesting despite public safeguarding intentions, the medical malpractice environment has created financial incentives (for lawyers, insurance schemes, etc.) for defensive practice. Ortashi et al. (2013) highlights that defensive practice is influenced by the court system which relies upon data (evidence of actions being taken) as opposed to clinician judgement, thus creating vicious cycles whereby health professionals feel safer from litigation by over-treating rather than undertreating patients. Additionally, research suggests the fear of litigation, not just the experience of litigation, can cause defensive practice (Pollard, 2011; Robertson & Thomson, 2016). Defensive practices have a detrimental effect on women's access to support and services for physiological births such as restricting services for vaginal birth after caesarean (Shorten, 2010), access to homebirth (Lee et al., 2016), access to waterbirth (Newnham, Elizabeth C. et al., 2015) etc. Therefore, a litigious culture alongside risk discourses and insurance policies required of institutions tends to super-value medicalised, technocratic practices, despite rhetorical commitments to evidence-based medicine and practice.

The politics of evidence-based medicine

Evidence-based medicine (EBM), evidence-based practice (EBP) and evidence-based healthcare (EBHC) are all terms used to depict a paradigm shift that began in the 1980s and proliferated in the 1990s (Berg, M., 2000). EBM was a move away from eminence-based practice i.e. custom, tradition, dogma and towards medical practice informed by scientific research (evidence) to achieve safe, more consistent and cost-effective outcomes (Greenhalgh, 2014; Weisz et al., 2007).[14] EBM was explicitly developed in opposition to excessive standardisation where population data was injudiciously applied to individuals and sought to develop methods to design, implement and assess scientific medical research (Sackett, 1997). Moreover, within its original conception, EBM explicitly centred on patient preference and clinical expertise to apply judgement to individual situations (Sackett, 1997) with a warning 'without clinical expertise, practice risks becoming tyrannized by external evidence ...' (p. 1).

EBM has been both 'heralded as one of the major advances in healthcare ... promising to revolutionise both policymaking and practice, and excoriated as a development reducing professionals to mindlessly (and soullessly) following recipe books' (p. 111) (Mullen & Streiner, 2004). Greenhalgh et al. (2014) describe seven key successes of EBM; the establishment of the Cochrane Collection that collate and summarise evidence from clinical trials, setting methodological and publication standards of research, building national and international infrastructures for developing and updating clinical practice guidelines, developing resources and courses for teaching critical appraisal and building the knowledge base for implementation and knowledge translation. Notwithstanding these successes, concerns have consistently highlighted an overemphasis on experimental knowledge has minimised the role of basic sciences,[15] the tacit knowledge of clinical expertise, and patient values (Wieringa, 2017).[16] Concerns regarding the applicability of population epidemiological studies to individual patients have been raised, particularly if professional discernment and patient preferences are not accounted for during decision-making (Kotaska, 2011; Rogers, 2004). Additional concerns regarding the misappropriation of the evidence-based quality mark by those with vested interests e.g., drug and biotechnology companies, financial (insurance companies), management and organisations have been raised (Greenhalgh, 2014; Ioannidis, 2017).

Other issues relate to what counts as evidence. Largely, modern science continues to perpetuate modernism from the 16th century. Modernism introduced secularisation and rational thought based on the belief that reality can be known via empirically testable scientific laws; therefore, nature and culture are seen separately (Wieringa, 2017). Modernism privileges rational facts, known as the Cartesian epistemology of differentiation, 'positivism', the analytical and disembodied (scientific) organisation of knowledge is privileged over tacit and situated experiences (Walsh, 2009). This has translated into a current hierarchy of evidence where randomised controlled trials (RCTs) are *perceived* as the 'gold standard' of collating evidence and informing clinical practice (Downe, 2010; Greenhalgh, 2015). However, the dominance of RCTs, risks a dogmatic approach[17] ignoring evidence from other sources such as the basic sciences, anatomy and physiology and may encourage research waste (Kennedy et al., 2018).

Given the vast costs involved with conducting an RCT, which may not be the appropriate methodology to answer a research question/problem, it is vital to reconsider this evidence hierarchy (Howick, 2011). In addition, recent thinking challenges the isolation of complex mechanisms to simplistic notions of what works (under these test conditions, with these particular research participants), that often fail to deliver the results attested to in the 'real world' (Downe, 2010; Greenhalgh, 2015; Wieringa, 2017).

Despite 40 years of challenging a simplified, linear approach to science (Illich, 1975; Kuhn, 1962), its dominance prevails. To which feminist researchers attribute a complex power structure of vested interest, dominance and subjugation. Challenging the assertion of positivism and rationality as value-free and objective, feminist scholars argue all research decisions are made from value judgements borne out of our worldview and positioning (Code, 1991; McHugh, 2015; Shuford, 2010). These values and world views are embedded throughout the research process maintaining and further entrenching gendered, class, and racial norms (McHugh, 2015; Shuford, 2010).[18] This point underpins the urgent necessity of intersectional representation throughout academia, healthcare and policy making (to name a few) as the only way to redress these imbalances. The marginalisation of women[19] occurs in numerous ways; the biomedical model of health ignores the social and political context of women's (ill) health, poor representation in research agendas, policy or within guideline development groups, the production of research i.e., agenda, inclusion (or rather exclusion), the methods used to analyse and synthesise, and the application of guidelines during clinical encounters (Doyal, 1979; Goldenberg, 2010; Rogers, 2004).

In maternity care, the politics of EBM is problematic and relates to how evidence/research is generated (who is asking what questions, from what position), what evidence counts (RCT evidence is dominant despite its inappropriateness for many research questions), what evidence is adopted and how quickly (aligning, or not, with the zeitgeist, influences adoption).[20] Evidence demonstrates most maternity-related research (and money invested) has focused on the pathologies of birth (Renfrew et al., 2014); revealing underlying values in favour of biomedicine and technologies. This has been at the expense of very little (comparatively) on the prevention of complications/pathologies and/or the support of women, which as Kennedy et al. (2018) argue, prevention is where the most gains are to be made. Even where there is strong evidence in favour of midwifery-led models of care, birthplace settings, and interventions such as water immersion for labour and birth,[21] wide-scale adoption is an ongoing challenge (Kennedy et al., 2018). Evidence for these midwifery-led interventions is frequently called into question and excessive demands are made for more research.[22] Yet, interventions aligned with the biotech model can be implemented in haste (Topçu & Brown, 2019), and once implemented, particularly at scale, 'de-implementing' or ceasing a practice is challenging (Grimshaw et al., 2020).[23] For example, despite 20 years of strong evidence refuting the benefits and demonstrating the harms, continuous electronic fetal monitoring (CEFM) is fortified within hospital care settings

(Kennedy et al., 2018; Small et al., 2020). Moreover, funding resources continue to be allocated to CEFM, arguably a significant waste of money (Sartwelle et al., 2017). CEFM is not the only example of the pre-eminence of biotech medicalised interventions in maternity care but provides a good illustration of the dominance of obstetric-led knowledge over midwifery-led knowledge.

Further concerns relate to the lack of evidence in maternity care in comparison to other specialities (Prusova et al., 2014), yet information for 'best practice' is embedded throughout national policies and hospital guidelines with significant influence on clinical practice and service-user experience. The Royal College of Obstetricians and Gynaecologists (RCOG) issues numerous maternity guideline recommendations and is a leading authority in the UK. However, when analysed to assess the evidence informing the recommendations, the 'Green Top Guidelines' were found to be lacking; of 1,682 individual recommendations, only 9–12% of the guidelines were based on best quality evidence (Prusova et al., 2014). In part, the lack of evidence has been attributed to ethical issues of conducting research with pregnant women (Blehar et al., 2013), and the acute nature of childbirth-related emergencies make trial design and implementation problematic (Vintzileos, 2009). However, issues of an overemphasis on pathology and medically informed research are argued as a bias against physiological, low-tech birth as previously described (Kennedy et al., 2018). Therefore, the production of research, the implementation and practice of EBM are not neutral, demonstrating that other political factors wield greater authority in maternity care.

Guideline-centred care, the crux of this research

This chapter has situated the key issues within UK maternity care, exploring the rhetoric versus the reality as related to midwifery care, physiological birth and the choice agenda. Drawing upon key sociocultural-political drivers, I examined possible reasons contributing to the tensions between rhetoric and reality. While not exhaustive, the medicalisation and institutionalisation of birth alongside risk, governance, litigation and defensive practice offer crucial insights to understanding the context of this study. These issues coalesce and can be captured as 'guideline-centred care' which is central to this research. A slow cultural shift changed clinical guidelines from helpful tools for busy practitioners, to 'rules to follow', whereby any deviation from the guideline must be justified. Or more commonly, must be defended. Due to governance and institutionalised practices, working 'within' the guidelines has become a proxy for so-called 'safe care'. Concepts of safety and its alignment with medico-institutional constructs of risk management are problematic. Crucially, guidelines are not infallible; they can be politically motivated, poorly developed, out of date, non-evidence based and not woman-centred. Birthing women and people do not have to legally conform to the guidelines however, research shows they can be steered, coerced and even bullied including punitive social services referrals should they not comply. Therefore, opting 'outside of guidelines', can be viewed as deviant or problematic, *despite* the centrality of individualised care within policy, legislation, international, national guidance and professional obligations. The next chapter explores how the employed midwives in this study navigated these issues and resisted succumbing to guideline-centred care to offer meaningful individualised and humanised care for those seeking alternative physiological birth care.

Notes

1 See Chapter 1 for discussion of 'normal' birth debate which appears to be most hotly contested in the UK.

2 Growing evidence has demonstrated the efficacy, safety, acceptability to women, and cost-effectiveness of non-OU birth settings (Brocklehurst, 2011; Burns et al., 2012; Hodnett et al., 2010). For healthy women at the onset of labour, birth outside of obstetric units is associated with greater levels of physiological births (Brocklehurst, 2011; Burns et al., 2012; Hodnett et al., 2010), women's satisfaction with their birth experience (McCourt et al., 2016; Olza et al., 2018), and midwives' sense of well-being and autonomy (McCourt et al., 2016). However, despite robust evidence and national clinical guidelines promoting women's access to non-OU settings (NICE, 2017), recent UK research demonstrates in 2020 only 2.4% women gave birth at home (a slight increase) (ONS, 2020) and approximately 14% in the UK gave birth in midwifery-led units (either AMU or FMU) (Walsh et al., 2018).

3 Homebirth and freestanding maternity unit closures escalated during the pandemic, with a few notable exceptions as demand for homebirth increased and a minority of services prioritised maintaining the services (Brigante et al., 2022; Romanis & Nelson, 2020).

4 In the UK, much emphasis is placed on the importance of woman or person-centred care, concepts wholly aligned with the human rights framework and supported by UK legislation. This legislation delineates women should have full bodily autonomy over their pregnancy and birthing decisions, assumes their mental capacity (unless proven otherwise), and includes the right to decline care, even where health professionals disagree with the decision. Therefore, woman/person-centred care, viewed within a legal lens, is an essential component of care provision; demands meaningful (and individualised) dialogue when care, treatments or interventions are offered; and where those are declined, those decisions are respected. Such dialogue (and subsequent caregiving responses) is how informed consent legislation, moral and professional obligations to preserve respect and dignity are actualised. And through the process of dialogue, a core aspect of caregiving, maternal autonomous decision-making is facilitated aka 'supported decision-making'.

5 There is much to say about the historical perspective of the rise of medical and institutional power, the purposeful discrediting of midwives, however, both Nadine Edwards (2005) and Elizabeth Newnham (2018) in their monographs have provided extensive analyses (among many others, I stand on the shoulders of many giants!). Therefore, to avoid repetition and to advance their work, here I try to bring those historical lenses to show how they influence and impact midwifery and birthing practices today.

6 The feminist argument that all choices are valid and bodily autonomy should be supported either way, for those seeking increased medical interventions and those who prefer less, is an ideal scenario. However, the actualisation of all women getting their needs met is deeply problematic, as the rest of the chapter will demonstrate the dominance of medicalised and institutionalised approaches frequently limits access to midwifery-led models of care and community births.

7 Also see (Newnham, E. et al., 2017; Roberts & Walsh, 2018).

8 Issues of midwives leaving the profession due to bullying is a consistent finding see also, (Curtis et al., 2006; Hunter et al., 2019; Leap, 1997).

 9 Other criticisms of guidelines include; the overwhelming number of guidelines rendering them inconvenient for busy professionals (Upshur, 2014), inaccessibility (The McDonnell Norms Group, 2006); flaws in their development (Prusova et al., 2014); oversimplification of complex illnesses (The McDonnell Norms Group, 2006); do not account for co-morbidities (Greenhalgh et al., 2015); lack of foresight regarding implementation procedures/efficacy (The McDonnell Norms Group, 2006); have become rules to follow which may not be beneficial to patient care (Berg, 2000; Downe, 2010; Greenhalgh et al., 2014; The McDonnell Norms Group, 2006).

10 Policies require mandatory compliance and are normally associated with terms of employment e.g., sickness, uniform, handwashing (Irving, 2014; RCM, 2022). Protocols, (processes or procedures), also require compliance but differ in that they are an agreed framework outlining the care that will be provided to women (or patients) in a designated are of practice (Irving, 2014; RCM, 2022). Examples include anaphylaxis management, eclampsia management, cardiac arrest, food handling on a ward etc.

11 All of the practices cited here have potential harms associated, therefore, when applied routinely, without a justifiable reason, can cause iatrogenic harms.

12 A key failing found in the Ockendon report were persistent 'cover ups', downgrading serious incidents, poorly conducted investigations, lack of Executive Board oversight or action, ignoring the families affected by failings and a lack of follow up or integration of the lessons learned (Ockendon, 2022). This is an example of self-protecting organisations at the expense of the wellbeing of the families suffering adverse events and outcomes.

13 Some cases have taken >10 years to reach a conclusion.

14 Obstetrics was famously awarded the 'wooden spoon' for its lack of evidence-based practice by Archie Cochrane, an early pioneer of EBM.

15 In maternity services these issues around the 'tyranny' of external evidence are seen when proponents of physiologically informed practices are required to continue to 'prove' physiology despite knowledge generated from the basic sciences, anatomy and physiological sciences. A prime example is with cord clamping (Niermeyer, 2015). Early cord clamping was a non-evidenced based intervention with proven harmful effects for the newborn. However, the onus has been on physiologists to 'prove' the harmful effects of early cord clamping, rather than proponents of early cord clamping required to prove its benefit. Change towards optimal cord clamping is occurring but slowly. (For extensive insights around cord clamping, see www.bloodtobaby.com.) Similar issues can be found throughout maternity care demonstrating the highly politicalised nature of knowledge generation and 'evidence-based practice'.

16 Also see (Goldenberg, 2010; Greenhalgh, 2014, 2015; Mullen & Streiner, 2004; Rogers, 2004; Upshur, 2014).

17 This was a heightened debate during COVID-19 where proponents of RCTs as the gold standard insisted mask wearing required an RCT. However, pragmatists resisted and challenged these calls through using the scientific knowledge at the time (Covid was airborne) and mask wearing was a low-risk intervention to reduce the spread (Greenhalgh, 2020).

18 Exposing the vast array of situations women are unaccounted for in science, health and technology is the recent book 'Invisible women: Exposing data bias in a world designed for men' (Criado-Perez, 2020).

19 All women have been subjected to marginalisation in the scientific project; however, such marginalisation is compounded for those in minoritised groups such as Black, Asian and Ethnic minority groups, disabled women, trans people and those in lower socioeconomic groups.

20 See (Davis-Floyd & Cheyney, 2009; Johanson et al., 2002; Kennedy et al., 2018; Kitzinger, 2005; Renfrew et al., 2014; Thomson & Crowther, 2019).

21 For the full range of potential midwifery-led interventions that have been found to be beneficial see Renfrew et al. (2014), as stated in Chapter 1, this seminal piece of work examined 13 meta-syntheses and 173 systematic reviews.

22 The evidence around homebirths, water births and continuity of carer are frequently called into question despite strong evidence in their favour, for the ongoing debates and criticisms, see (ACOG, 2011; ACOG, 2014; Ockendon, 2022; Wax et al., 2010).
23 Examples included (but not limited to) induction and/or augmentation with syntocinon, prophylactic antibiotics, fetal blood sampling, episiotomies, early cord clamping. Also see a blog I wrote about de-implementing an intervention called 'fresh ears' that was introduced without evidence and with potential harms (Feeley, 2020).

References

Abalos, E., Oladapo, O., Chamillard, M., DÃaz, V., Pasquale, J., Bonet, M., Souza, J., & GÃ¼lmezoglu, A. (2018). Duration of spontaneous labour in low-risk women with normal perinatal outcomes: A systematic review. *European Journal of Obstetrics, Gynecology, and Reproductive Biology*, 223, 123–132. doi: 10.1016/j.ejogrb.2018.02.026

Abbasi, K. (2022). A system reset for the campaign against too much medicine. *BMJ*, 377, o1466. https://www.bmj.com/content/377/bmj.o1466

ACOG. (2011). ACOG committee opinion No. 476: Planned home birth. *Obstetrics and Gynecology*, 117, 425–428.

ACOG. (2014). Immersion in water during labor and delivery: Committee's opinion 679. *Contemporary Obstetrics & Gynecology*, 59(4). https://www.acog.org/clinical/clinical-guidance/committee-opinion/articles/2016/11/immersion-in-water-during-labor-and-delivery

Alaszewski, A., Harrison, L., & Manthorpe, J. (1998). *Risk, Health and Welfare*. Open University Press.

Alexander, C. R., & Bogossian, F. (2018). Midwives and clinical investigation: A review of the literature. *Women and Birth: Journal of the Australian College of Midwives*, 31(6), 442–452. doi: 10.1016/j.wombi.2018.02.003

Annandale, E., & Clark, J. (1996). What is gender? Feminist theory and the sociology of human reproduction. *Sociology on Health & Illness*, 18(1), 17–44.

Arulkumaran, S. (2010). Clinical governance and standards in UK maternity care to improve quality and safety. *Midwifery*, 26(5), 485–487. doi: 10.1016/j.midw.2010.08.002

Beck, U. (1992). *Risk Society: Towards a New Modernity*. Sage.

Beckett, K. (2005). Choosing Cesarean: Feminism and the politics of childbirth in the United States. *Feminist Theory*, 6(3), 251–275. doi: 10.1177/1464700105057363

Beech, B. (2016). Homebirth and the regulator: An abrogation of responsibility. *British Journal of Midwifery*, 24(12), 879–881. doi: 10.12968/bjom.2016.24.12.879

Behruzi, R., Hatem, M., Goulet, L., Fraser, W., & Misago, C. (2013). Understanding childbirth practices as an organizational cultural phenomenon: A conceptual framework. *BMC Pregnancy and Birth*, 13(205). doi: 10.1186/1471-2393-13-205

Berg, L., Thomson, G., Jonge, A. D., Balaam, M., Moncrieff, G., Topalidou, A., & Downe, S. (2022). 'Never waste a crisis': A commentary on the COVID-19 pandemic as a driver for innovation in maternity care. *BJOG: An International Journal of Obstetrics & Gynaecology*, 129(1), 3–8. doi: 10.1111/1471-0528.16996

Berg, M. (2000). Guidelines, professionals and the production of objectivity: Standardisation and the professionalism of insurance medicine. *Sociology of Health and Illness*, 22(6), 765–791.

Birth choice UK/Which? (2015). Retrieved from http://www.birthchoiceuk.com/

Birthrights. (2013). *The Dignity Survey 2013: Women's and Midwives' Experiences of UK Maternity Care*. London: Birthrights. https://birthrights.org.uk/wp-content/uploads/2013/10/Birthrights-Dignity-Survey-1.pdf

Birthrights. (2018). *Maternal request Caesarean*. Birthrights. https://www.birthrights.org.uk/campaigns-research/maternal-request-caesarean/

Birthrights. (2022a). *Inquiry on racial injustice in maternity care: Terms of reference*. https://www.birthrights.org.uk/wp-content/uploads/2021/03/Inquiry-on-racial-injustice-terms-of-reference-FINAL.pdf

Birthrights. (2022b). *Systemic racism, not broken bodies An inquiry into racial injustice and human rights in UK maternity care.* https://www.birthrights.org.uk/wp-content/uploads/2022/05/Birthrights-inquiry-systemic-racism_exec-summary_May-22-web.pdf

Blaylock, R., Trickey, H., Sanders, J., & Murphy, C. (2022). WRISK voices: A mixed-methods study of women's experiences of pregnancy-related public health advice and risk messages in the UK. *Midwifery*, 113, 103433. doi: 10.1016/j.midw.2022.103433

Blehar, M., Spong, C., Grady, C., Goldkind, S., Sahin, L., & Clayton, J. (2013). Enrolling pregnant women: Issues in clinical research. *Women's Health Issues: Official Publication of the Jacobs Institute of Women's Health*, 23(1), e39–e45. doi: 10.1016/j.whi.2012.10.003

Brigante, L., Morelli, A., Jokinen, M., Plachcinski, R., & Rowe, R. (2022). Impact of the COVID-19 pandemic on midwifery-led service provision in the United Kingdom in 2020–21: Findings of three national surveys. *Midwifery*, 112, 103390. doi: 10.1016/j.midw.2022.103390

Brocklehurst, P. (2011). Perinatal and maternal outcomes by planned place of birth for healthy women with low risk pregnancies: The birthplace in England national prospective cohort study. *BMJ*, 343, d7400. doi: 10.1136/bmj.d7400

Brubaker, S., & Dillaway, H. (2009). Medicalization, natural childbirth and birthing experiences. *Sociology Compass*, 3(1), 31–48.

Budgeon, S. (2015). Individualized femininity and feminist politics of choice. *European Journal of Women's Studies*, 22(3), 303–318. doi: 10.1177/1350506815576602

Burns, E. E., Boulton, M. G., Cluett, E., Cornelius, V. R., & Smith, L. A. (2012). Characteristics, interventions, and outcomes of women who used a birthing pool: A prospective observational study. *Birth*, 39(3), 192–202. doi: 10.1111/j.1523-536X.2012.00548.x

Cahill, H. (2000). Male appropriation and medicalization of childbirth: An historical analysis. *Journal of Advancing Nursing*, 33(3); 334–342.

Campbell, R., & Porter, S. (1997). Feminist theory and the sociology of childbirth: A response to Ellen Annandale and Judith Clark. *Sociology of Health & Illness*, 19(3), 348–358.

Cidro, J., Bach, R., Frohlick, J. (2020). Canada's forced birth travel: towards feminist indigenous reproductive mobilities. *Mobilities*, 15(2), 173–187, DOI: 10.1080/17450101.2020.1730611

Clesse, C., Lighezzolo-Alnot, J., de Lavergne, S., Hamlin, S., & Scheffler, M. (2018). The evolution of birth medicalisation: A systematic review. *Midwifery*, 66, 161–167. doi: 10.1016/j.midw.2018.08.003

Code, L. (1991). *What Can She Know? Feminist Theory and the Construction of Knowledge*. Cornell University Press.

Criado-Perez, C. (2020). *Invisible Women: Exposing the Gender Bias Women Face Every Day*. Vintage.

Curtis, P., Ball, L., & Kirkham, M. (2006). Why do midwives leave? (not) being the kind of midwife you want to be. *British Journal of Midwifery*, 14(1), 27–31.

Dahlen, H. (2010). Undone by fear? Deluded by trust? *Midwifery*, 26(2), 156–162. doi: 10.1016/j.midw.2009.11.008

Dahlen, H. G., & Caplice, S. (2014). What do midwives fear? *Women Birth*, 27(4), 266–270. doi: 10.1016/j.wombi.2014.06.008

Davis-Floyd, R., & Cheyney, M. (2009). Birth and the big bad wolf: An evolutionary perspective. In H. Selin & P. Stone (Eds.), *Childbirth across Cultures: Ideas and Practices of Pregnancy, Childbirth, and the Postpartum* (pp. 1–22). Springer.

De Vries, R. (1984). "Humanizing" childbirth: The discovery and implementation of bonding theory. *International Journal of Health Services: Planning, Administration, Evaluation*, 14(1), 89–104.

Dekker, S. W. A., & Nyce, J. M. (2012). Cognitive engineering and the moral theology and witchcraft of cause. *Cognition, Technology & Work*, 14(3), 207–212. doi: 10.1007/s10111-011-0203-6

Department, O. H. (1970). *The Peel Report*. London: HMSO.

DH. (1993). *Changing Childbirth*. London: Department of Health.

DH. (2007). *Maternity Matters. Choice, Access and Continuity of Care in a Safe Service*. London: Department of Health.

DH. (2010). *Midwifery 2020: Delivering Expectations*. Cambridge: Jill Rogers Associates.

Dodwell, M. (2012). *Normal Birth Rates for England*. London: NCT. Retrieved from https://www.nct.org.uk/sites/default/files/related_documents/Dodwell%20Normal%20birth%20rates%20for%20England%20PerspSept12%20p16-17.pdf

Downe, S. (2010). Beyond evidence-based medicine: Complexity and stories of maternity care. *Journal of Evaluation in Clinical Practice*, 16(1), 232–237. doi: 10.1111/j.1365-2753.2009.01357.x

Downe, S., & Finlayson, K. (2016). *Interventions in Normal Labour and Birth*. London: Royal College of Midwives. SDowne@uclan.ac.uk

Downe, S., Finlayson, K., & Fleming, A. (2010). Creating a collaborative culture in maternity care. *Journal of Midwifery & Women's Health*, 55(3), 250–254. doi: 10.1016/j.jmwh.2010.01.004

Downe, S., Finlayson, K., Oladapo, O., Bonet, M., & GÂlmezoglu, A. (2018). What matters to women during childbirth: A systematic qualitative review. 13(4). doi: 10.1371/journal.pone.0194906

Downe, S., & McCourt, C. (2004). From being to becoming: Reconstructing childbirth knowledges. In S. Downe (Ed.), *Normal Birth, Evidence and Debate* (pp. 3–24). Elsevier.

Doyal, L. (1979). *The Political Economy of Health*. Pluto Press.

Edwards, N. (2005). *Birthing Autonomy: Women's Experiences of Planning Home Births*. Routledge.

Edwards, N., Murphy-Lawless, J., Kirkham, M., & Davies, S. (2011). Attacks on midwives, attacks on women's choices. *Association for Improvements in the Maternity Services*, 23(3). http://www.aims.org.uk/Journal/Vol23No3/attacks.htm#38

England, N. (2017). *Implementing Better Births: Continuity of Carer*. NHS England. https://www.england.nhs.uk/wp-content/uploads/2017/12/implementing-better-births.pdf

Euro-Peristat Project. (2018). *European Perinatal Health Report. Core Indicators of the Health and Care of Pregnant Women and Babies in Europe in 2015*. Paris: Euro-Peristat Project.

Feeley, C. (2020). De-implementing 'fresh ears'. https://www.all4maternity.com/de-implementing-fresh-ears/

Feeley, C., & Thomson, G. (2016). Tensions and conflicts in 'choice': Womens' experiences of freebirthing in the UK. *Midwifery*, 41, 16–21. doi: 10.1016/j.midw.2016.07.014

Fenwick, J., Hammond, A., Raymond, J., Smith, R., Gray, J., Foureur, M., Homer, C., & Symon, A. (2012). Surviving, not thriving: A qualitative study of newly qualified midwivesâ€™ experience of their transition to practice. 21(13), 2054–2063. doi: 10.1111/j.1365-2702.2012.04090.x

Foucault, M. (1973). *The Birth of a Clinic: An Archaeology of Medical Perception.* Tavistock.

Gillen, P., Sinclair, M., & Kernohan, G. (2008). *The Nature and Manifestations of Bullying in Midwifery.* Ulster: University of Ulster. http://www.thewisehippo.com/wp-content/uploads/2016/04/University_of-Ulster_The_nature_and_manifestations_of_bullying_in_midwifery_Research_Summary.pdf

Goldenberg, M. (2010). Perspectives on evidence-based healthcare for women. *Journal of Women's Health*, 19(7), 1235–1238. doi: 10.1089/jwh.2009.1680

Goldkuhl, L., Dellenborg, L., Berg, M., Wijk, H., & Nilsson, C. (2022). The influence and meaning of the birth environment for nulliparous women at a hospital-based labour ward in Sweden: An ethnographic study. *Women and Birth*, 35(4), e337–e347. doi: 10.1016/j.wombi.2021.07.005

Greenhalgh, T. (2014). Evidence based medicine: A movement in crisis? *BMJ*, 348:g3725 https://doi.org/10.1136/bmj.g3725

Greenhalgh, T. (2015). Six biases against patients and carers in evidence-based medicine. *BMC Medicine*, 13(200). https://doi.org/10.1186/s12916-015-0437-x

Greenhalgh, T. (2020). Face coverings for the public: Laying straw men to rest. *Journal of Evaluation in Clinical Practice*, 26(4), 1070–1077. doi: 10.1111/jep.13415

Griffith, R., & Tengnah, C. (2010). *Law and Professional Issues in Midwifery (Transforming Midwifery Practice Series).* Learning Matters Ltd.

Grimshaw, J. M., Patey, A. M., Kirkham, K. R., Hall, A., Dowling, S. K., Rodondi, N., Ellen, M., Kool, T., van Dulmen, S. A., Kerr, E. A., Linklater, S., Levinson, W., & Bhatia, R. S. (2020). De-implementing wisely: Developing the evidence base to reduce low-value care. *BMJ Quality & Safety*, 29(5), 409–417. doi: 10.1136/bmjqs-2019-010060

Haslem, L. (2011). Monstrous issues: The uterus as riddle in early modern texts. In A. Mangham, & G. Depledge (Eds.), *The Female Body in Medicine and Literature* (pp. 34–50). Liverpool University Press.

Healy, S., Humphreys, E., & Kennedy, C. (2016). Can maternity care move beyond risk? Implications for midwifery as a profession. *British Journal of Midwifery*, 24(3), 203–209. doi: 10.12968/bjom.2016.24.3.203

Hodnett, E. D., Downe, S., & Walsh, D. (2012). Alternative versus conventional institutional settings for birth. *Cochrane Database of Systematic Reviews*. doi: 10.1002/14651858. CD000012.pub4

Hodnett, E. D., Downe, S., Walsh, D., & Weston, J. (2010). Alternative versus conventional institutional settings for birth. *Cochrane Database of Systematic Reviews*. doi: 10.1002/14651858.cd000012.pub3

Howick, J. (2011). *The Philosophy of Evidence-based Medicine.* Wiley-Blackwell.

Hunt, S., & Symonds, A. (1995). *The Social Meaning of Midwifery.* Macmillan.

Hunter, B., Fenwick, J., Sidebotham, M., & Henley, J. (2019). Midwives in the United Kingdom: Levels of burnout, depression, anxiety and stress and associated predictors. doi: 7910.1016/j.midw.2019.08.008

Hunter, B., Henley, J., Fenwick, J., Sidebotham, M., & Pallant, J. (2018). *Work, Health and Emotional Lives of Midwives in the United Kingdom: The UK WHELM Study.* Cardiff: Cardiff University. https://www.rcm.org.uk/sites/default/files/UK%20WHELM%20REPORT%20final%20180418-May.pdf

Hunter, B., & Segrott, J. (2014). Renegotiating inter-professional boundaries in maternity care: Implementing a clinical pathway for normal labour. *Sociology of Health & Illness*, 36(5), 719–737. doi: 10.1111/1467-9566.12096

Illich, I. (1975). *The Medicalization of Life*. London: Society for the Study of Medical Ethics.

Ioannidis, J. (2017). Hijacked evidence-based medicine: Stay the course and throw the pirates overboard. *Journal of Clinical Epidemiology*, 84, 11–13. doi: 10.1016/j.jclinepi.2017.02.001

Irving, A. (2014). *Policies and Procedures for Healthcare Organizations: A Risk Management Perspective*. https://www.psqh.com/analysis/policies-and-procedures-for-healthcare-organizations-a-risk-management-perspective/#

Johannessen, L. (2017). Beyond guidelines: Discretionary practice in face-to-face triage nursing. *Sociology of Health & Illness*, 39(7) 1180-1194.

Johanson, R., Newburn, M., & Macfarlane, A. (2002). Has the medicalisation of childbirth gone too far? *BMJ*, 324(7342), 892–895. doi: 10.1136/bmj.324.7342.892

Keedle, H., Schmied, V., Burns, E., & Dahlen, H. G. (2015). Women's reasons for, and experiences of, choosing a homebirth following a caesarean section. *BMC Pregnancy and Childbirth*, 15(1), 206. doi: 10.1186/s12884-015-0639-4

Kennedy, H. P., Cheyney, M., Dahlen, H. G., Downe, S., Foureur, M. J., Homer, C. S. E., Jefford, E., McFadden, A., Michel-Schuldt, M., Sandall, J., Soltani, H., Speciale, A. M., Stevens, J., Vedam, S., & Renfrew, M. J. (2018). Asking different questions: A call to action for research to improve the quality of care for every woman, every child. *Birth*, 45(3), 222–231. doi: 10.1111/birt.12361

King's Fund. (2012). *Improving Safety in Maternity: Communication*. https://www.kingsfund.org.uk/sites/default/files/field/field_related_document/Improving-safety-in-maternity-services-communication1.pdf

Kirkham, M. (2003). A 'cycle of empowerment': The enabling culture of birth centres. *The Practising Midwife*, 6(11), 12–15.

Kirkup, B. (2015). *The Report of the Morecambe Bay Investigation*. Morecambe Bay Investigation. https://assets.publishing.service.gov.uk/government/uploads/system/uploads/attachment_data/file/408480/47487_MBI_Accessible_v0.1.pdf

Kitzinger, S. (2005). *The Politics of Birth*. Elsevier.

Klein, M., Sakala, C., Simkin, P., Davis-Floyd, R., Rooks, J., & Pincus, J. (2006). Why do women go along with this stuff? *Birth*, 33(3), 245–250. doi: 10.1111/j.1523-536X.2006.00110.x

Koerber, A., Arduser, L., Bennett, J., Kolodziejski, L., Sastry, S., & Strait, P. (2015). Risk and vulnerable, medicalized bodies. *Poroi*, 11(1), 1–9.

Kotaska, A. (2011). Guideline-centered care: A two-edged sword. *Birth*, 38(2), 97–98. doi: 10.1111/j.1523-536X.2011.00469.x

Kuhn, T. (1962). *The Structure of Scientific Revolutions*. University of Chicago Press.

Leap, N. (1997). Making sense of horizontal violence in midwifery. *British Journal of Midwifery*, 5(11), 689. doi: 10.12968/bjom.1997.5.11.689

Lee, S., Ayers, S., & Holden, D. (2016). Risk perception and choice of place of birth in women with high-risk pregnancies: A qualitative study. *Midwifery*, 38, 49–54. doi: 10.1016/j.midw.2016.03.008

Levy, V. (1999). Protective steering: A grounded theory study of the processes by which midwives facilitate informed choices during pregnancy. *Journal of Advanced Nursing*, 29(1), 104–112.

Maher, J. (2008). Progressing through labour and delivery: Birth time and women's experiences. *Women's Studies International Forum*, 31(2), 129–137.

Martin, E. (1987). *The Woman in the Body: A Cultural Analysis of Reproduction*. Milton Keynes: Open University Press.

Maturo, A. (2012). Medicalization: Current concept and future directions in a bionic society. *Mens Sana Monographs*, 10(1):122–133. doi: 10.4103/0973-1229.91587

MBRRACE-UK. (2021). *Saving Lives, Improving Mothers' Care Lessons Learned to Inform Maternity Care from the UK and Ireland Confidential Enquiries into Maternal Deaths and Morbidity 2017–19.* Oxford: National Perinatal Epidemiology Unit, University of Oxford. https://www.npeu.ox.ac.uk/assets/downloads/mbrrace-uk/reports/maternal-report-2021/MBRRACE-UK_Maternal_Report_2021_-_FINAL_-_WEB_VERSION.pdf

McAra-Couper, J., Jones, M., & Smythe, L. (2011). Caesarean-section, my body, my choice: The construction of 'informed choice' in relation to intervention in childbirth. *Feminism & Psychology,* 22(1), 81–97. doi: 10.1177/0959353511424369

McCourt, C., & Dykes, F. (2009). From traditional to modernity: Time and childbirth in historical perspective. In C. McCourt (Ed.), *Childbirth, Midwifery and Concepts of Time* (pp. 17–36). Berghahn Books.

McCourt, C., Rance, S., Rayment, J., & Sandall, J. (2011). *Birthplace Qualitative Organisational Case Studies: How Maternity Care Systems May Affect the Provision of Care in Different Birth Settings. Birthplace in England Research Programme.* Final report part 6. IHR Service Delivery and Organisation programme. https://openaccess.city.ac.uk/id/eprint/3641/1/Birthplace%20Case%20Studies%20SDO_FR6_08-1604-140_V01.pdf

McCourt, C., Rayment, J., Rance, S., & Sandall, J. (2016). Place of birth and concepts of wellbeing. *Journal for Applied Anthropology in Policy and Practice,* 23(3), 17–29.

McDonald, R., Waring, J., Harrison, S., Walshe, K., & Boaden, R. (2005). Rules and guidelines in clinical practice: A qualitative study in operating theatres of doctors' and nurses' views. *BMJ Quality & Safety,* 14(4), 290–294. doi: 10.1136/qshc.2005.013912

McHugh, N. (2015). *The Limits of Knowledge: Generating Pragmatist Feminist Cases for Situated Knowing.* State University of New York Press.

McMahon, M., & Ashworth, E. (2020). *Social Care Referrals: Lifting the Lid.* https://www.all4maternity.com/social-care-referrals-lifting-the-lid/

Mullen, E., & Streiner, D. (2004). The evidence for and against evidence-based practice. *Brief Treatment and Crisis Intervention,* 4(2), 111–121. doi: 10.1093/brief-treatment/mhh009

National Health Service, Litigation Authority. (2016). *NHS Litigation Authority Annual Report and Accounts 2015/16.* London: National Health Service Litigation Authority.

Naylor Smith, J., Taylor, B., Shaw, K., Hewison, A., & Kenyon, S. (2018). 'I didn't think you were allowed that, they didn't mention that.' A qualitative study exploring women's perceptions of home birth. *BMC Pregnancy and Childbirth,* 18(1), 105. doi: 10.1186/s12884-018-1733-1

Newnham, E. (2014). Birth control: Power/knowledge in the politics of birth. *Health Sociology Review,* 23(3), 254–268. doi: 10.1080/14461242.2014.11081978

Newnham, E., & Kirkham, M. (2019). Beyond autonomy: Care ethics for midwifery and the humanization of birth. *Nursing Ethics,* 26(7–8), 2147–2157. doi: 10.1177/0969733018819119

Newnham, E., McKellar, L., & Pincombe, J. (2017). Paradox of the institution: Findings from a hospital labour ward ethnography. *BMC Pregnancy and Childbirth,* 17(1). doi: 10.1186/s12884-016-1193-4

Newnham, E., McKellar, L., & Pincombe, J. (2018). Introduction. In E. Newnham, L. McKellar & J. Pincombe (Eds.), *Towards the Humanisation of Birth: A Study of Epidural Analgesia and Hospital Birth Culture* (pp. 1–15). Palgrave Macmillan.

Newnham, E., McKellar, L., & Pincombe, J. (2015). Documenting risk: A comparison of policy and information pamphlets for using epidural or water in labour. *Women Birth,* 28(3), 221–227. doi: 10.1016/j.wombi.2015.01.012

NHS Digital. (2018). *NHS Maternity Statistics, England 2017–18.* digital.nhs.uk. https://digital.nhs.uk/data-and-information/publications/statistical/nhs-maternity-statistics/2017-18

NHS Digital. (2021). *NHS Maternity Statistics, England – 2020–21.* digital.nhs.uk. https://digital.nhs.uk/data-and-information/publications/statistical/nhs-maternity-statistics/2020-21#top

NHS England. (2016). *Better Births: Improving Outcomes of Maternity Services in England. A Five Year Forward View for maternity care.* https://www.england.nhs.uk/wp-content/uploads/2016/02/national-maternity-review-report.pdf

NHS England and Improvement. (2021). *Personalised Care and Support Planning Guidance: Guidance for Local Maternity Systems.* London: NHS England. https://www.england.nhs.uk/wp-content/uploads/2021/03/B0423-personalised-care-and-support-planning-guidance-for-lms.pdf

NICE. (2017). *Intrapartum Care for Healthy Women and Babies.* NICE. https://www.nice.org.uk/guidance/cg190/resources/intrapartum-care-for-healthy-women-and-babies-pdf-35109866447557

NICE. (2021). *Antenatal Care NICE Guideline [NG201].* London: National Institute for Healthcare and Excellence. https://www.nice.org.uk/guidance/ng201

Niermeyer, S. (2015). A physiologic approach to cord clamping: Clinical issues. *Maternal Health, Neonatology and Perinatology,* 1(1), 21. doi: 10.1186/s40748-015-0022-5

NMPA. (2019). National Maternity and Perinatal Audit: Clinical Report 2019. Based on births in NHS maternity services between 1 April 2016 and 31 March 2017. RCOG, London. https://maternityaudit.org.uk/FilesUploaded/NMPA%20Clinical%20Report%202019.pdf

NMPA Project Team. (2022). *National Maternity and Perinatal Audit Clinical Report 2022 Based on Births in NHS Maternity Services in England and Wales between 1 April 2018 and 31 March 2019.* London: RCOG. https://maternityaudit.org.uk/FilesUploaded/Ref%20336%20NMPA%20Clinical%20Report_2022.pdf

Oakley, A. (1986). *The Captured Womb: History of the Medical Care of Pregnant Women.* Wiley-Blackwell.

Ockendon, D. (2022). *Findings, Conclusions and Essential Actions from the Independent Review of Maternity Services at the Shrewsbury and Telford Hospital NHS Trust.* London: HH Associates Ltd. https://www.gov.uk/government/publications/final-report-of-the-ockenden-review

Olza, I., Leahy-Warren, P., Benyamini, Y., Kazmierczak, M., Karlsdottir, S., Spyridou, A., Crespo-Mirasol, E., TakÃjcs, L., Hall, P., Murphy, M., Jonsdottir, S., Downe, S., & Nieuwenhuijze, M. (2018). Women's psychological experiences of physiological childbirth: A meta-synthesis. *BMJ Open,* 8(10). doi: 10.1136/bmjopen-2017-020347

ONS. (2020). *Birth Characteristics in England and Wales: 2020.* https://www.ons.gov.uk/peoplepopulationandcommunity/birthsdeathsandmarriages/livebirths/bulletins/birthcharacteristicsinenglandandwales/2020#place-of-birth

Ortashi, O., Virdee, J., Hassan, R., Mutrynowski, T., & Abu-Zidan, F. (2013). The practice of defensive medicine among hospital doctors in the United Kingdom. 14(1). doi: 10.1186/1472-6939-14-42

Plested, M., & Kirkham, M. (2016). Risk and fear in the lived experience of birth without a midwife. *Midwifery,* 38, 29–34. doi: 10.1016/j.midw.2016.02.009

Pollard, K. (2011). How midwives' discursive practices contribute to the maintenance of the status quo in English maternity care. *Midwifery,* 27(5), 612–619.

Prusova, K., Churcher, L., Tyler, A., & Lokugamage, A. (2014). Royal college of obstetricians and gynaecologists guidelines: How evidence-based are they? 34(8), 706–711. doi: 10.3109/01443615.2014.920794

RCM. (2011). *The Royal College of Midwives Survey of Midwives' Current Thinking about Homebirth*. London: Royal College of Midwives.

RCM. (2022). *Care Outside Guidance Caring for Those Women Seeking Choices That Fall Outside Guidance*. London: Royal College of Midwives. https://www.rcm.org.uk/media/5941/care_outside_guidance.pdf

Reed, R., Sharman, R., & Inglis, C. (2017). Women's descriptions of childbirth trauma relating to care provider actions and interactions. *BMC Pregnancy and Childbirth*. doi: 1710.1186/s12884-016-1197-0

Reiger, K., & Morton, C. (2012). Standardizing or individualizing? A critical analysis of the "discursive imaginaries" shaping maternity care reform. *International Journal of Childbirth*, (3), 173–186. doi: 10.1891/0886-6708.2.3.173

Reitsma, A., Simioni, J., Brunton, G., Kaufman, K., & Hutton, E. K. (2020). Maternal outcomes and birth interventions among women who begin labour intending to give birth at home compared to women of low obstetrical risk who intend to give birth in hospital: A systematic review and meta-analyses. *The Lancet*, 5(21), 100319. doi: 10.1016/j.eclinm.2020.100319

Renfrew, M., McFadden, A., Bastos, M., Campbell, J., Channon, A., Cheung, N., Silva, D., Downe, S., Kennedy, H., Malata, A., McCormick, F., Wick, L., & Declercq, E. (2014). Midwifery and quality care: Findings from a new evidence-informed framework for maternal and newborn care. *Lancet*, 384(9948), 1129–1145. doi: 10.1016/S0140-6736(14)60789-3

Riessman, C. (1983). Women and medicalization: A new perspective. *Social Policy*, 14(1), 3–18.

Roberts, J., & Walsh, D. (2018). Babies come when they are ready: Women's experiences of resisting the medicalisation of prolonged pregnancy. 0(0). doi: 10.1177/0959353518799386

Robertson, J. H., & Thomson, A. M. (2016). An exploration of the effects of clinical negligence litigation on the practice of midwives in England: A phenomenological study. *Midwifery*, 33, 55–63. doi: 10.1016/j.midw.2015.10.005

Rogers, W. (2004). Evidence-based medicine and women: Do the principles and practice of EBM further women's health? *Bioethics*, 18(1), 50–71. doi: 10.1111/j.1467-8519.2004.00378.x

Rogers, W., Entwistle, V., & Carter, S. (2019). Risk, overdiagnosis and ethical justifications. *Health Care Analysis*, 27(4), 231–248. doi: 10.1007/s10728-019-00369-7

Romanis, E. C., & Nelson, A. (2020). Homebirthing in the United Kingdom during COVID-19. *Medical Law International*, 20(3), 183–200. doi: 10.1177/0968533220955224

Russell, K. (2011). Struggling to get into the pool room? A Critical discourse analysis of labor ward midwives' experiences of water birth. *International Journal of Childbirth*, 1, 52–60. doi: 10.1891/2156-5287.1.1.52

Sackett, D. (1997). Evidence-based medicine. *Seminars in Perinatology*, 21(1), 3–5.

Sandall, J., Soltani, H., Gates, S., Shennan, A., & Devane, D. (2016). Midwife-led continuity models versus other models of care for childbearing women. *Cochrane Database of Systematic Reviews*, (4). doi: 10.1002/14651858.CD004667.pub5

Sanders, R. A., & Crozier, K. (2018). How do informal information sources influence women's decision-making for birth? A meta-synthesis of qualitative studies. *BMC Pregnancy and Childbirth*, 18(1), 21. doi: 10.1186/s12884-017-1648-2

Sartwelle, T. P., Johnston, J. C., & Arda, B. (2017). A half century of electronic fetal monitoring and bioethics: Silence speaks louder than words. *Maternal Health, Neonatology and Perinatology*, 3, 21. doi: 10.1186/s40748-017-0060-2

Scamell, M. (2014). 'She can't come here!' Ethics and the case of birth centre admission policy in the UK. *Journal of Medical Ethics*, 40(12), 813–816.

Scamell, M. (2016). The fear factor of risk – clinical governance and midwifery talk and practice in the UK. *Midwifery*, 38, 14–20. doi: 10.1016/j.midw.2016.02.010

Scamell, M., & Alaszewski, A. (2012). Fateful moments and the categorisation of risk: Midwifery practice and the ever-narrowing window of normality during childbirth. 14(2), 207–221. doi: 10.1080/13698575.2012.661041

Shallow, H. (2013). Deviant mothers and midwives: supporting VBAC with women as real partners in decision making. *Essentially MIDIRS*, 4(1), 17–21.

Sheikh, S., Ganesaratnam, I., & Jan, H. (2013). The birth of forceps. 4(7), 1–4. doi: 10.1177/2042533313478412

Sheridan, V. (2010). Organisational culture and routine midwifery practice on labour ward: Implications for mother-baby contact. *Evidence Based Midwifery*, 8(3), 76–84.

Shorten, A. (2010). Bridging the gap between mothers and medicine: "New insights" from the NIH Consensus Conference on VBAC. *Birth*, 37(3), 181–183. doi: 10.1111/j.1523-536X.2010.00404.x

Shuford, A. (2010). *Feminist Epistemology and American Pragmatism: Dewey and Quine*. Continuum International Publishing Group.

Skrondal, T. F., Bache-Gabrielsen, T., & Aune, I. (2020). All that I need exists within me: A qualitative study of nulliparous Norwegian women's experiences with planned home birth. *Midwifery*, 86, 102705. doi: 10.1016/j.midw.2020.102705

Small, K. A., Sidebotham, M., Fenwick, J., & Gamble, J. (2020). Intrapartum cardiotocograph monitoring and perinatal outcomes for women at risk: Literature review. *Women and Birth*, 33(5), 411–418. doi: 10.1016/j.wombi.2019.10.002

Smith, A., & Dixon, A. (2008). *Health Care Professionals' Views about Safety in Maternity Services*. London: King's Fund. https://www.kingsfund.org.uk/sites/default/files/pro_evidence.pdf

Stacey, M. (1988). *The Sociology of Health and Healing*. Unwin Hyman.

Symon, A. (2000). Litigation and defensive clinical practice: Quantifying the problem. *Midwifery*, 16(1), 8–14. doi: 10.1054/midw.1999.0181

The McDonnell Norms Group (2006). Enhancing the use of clinical guidelines: A social norms perspective. *Journal of the American College of Surgeons*, 202(5), 826–836.

Thomson, G., Feeley, C., Hall Moran, V., Downe, S., & Oladapo, O. (2019). Women's experiences of pharmacological and non-pharmacological pain relief methods for labour and childbirth: A qualitative systematic review. *BMC Reproductive Health*, 30; 16(1), 71. doi: 10.1186/s12978-019-0735-4

Thomson, G., & Crowther, S. (2019). Phenomenology as a political position within maternity care. *Nursing Philosophy: An International Journal for Healthcare Professionals*, 20(4), e12275. doi: 10.1111/nup.12275

Thwaites, R. (2017). Making a choice or taking a stand? Choice feminism, political engagement and the contemporary feminist movement. *Feminist Theory*, 18(1), 55–68. doi: 10.1177/1464700116683657

Topçu, S., & Brown, P. (2019). The impact of technology on pregnancy and childbirth: Creating and managing obstetrical risk in different cultural and socio-economic contexts. *Health, Risk & Society*, 21(3–4), 89–99. doi: 10.1080/13698575.2019.1649922

Upshur, R. (2014). Do clinical guidelines still make sense? *Annals of Family Medicine*, 2(3): 202–203. doi: 10.1370/afm.1654 van Teijlingen, E. (2005). A critical analysis of the medical model as used in the study of pregnancy and childbirth. *Sociological Research Online*, 10(2), 1–16.

Vintzileos, A. (2009). Evidence-based compared with reality-based medicine in obstetrics. *Obstetrics and Gynecology*, 113(6), 1335–1340. doi: 10.1097/AOG.0b013e3181a11b99

Walsh, D. (2006). Subverting the assembly-line: Childbirth in a free-standing birth centre. *Social Science & Medicine* 62(6), 1330–1340. doi: 10.1016/j.socscimed.2005.08.013

Walsh, D. (2007). *Improving Maternity Services: Small Is Beautiful - Lessons from a Birth Centre*. Radcliffe Publishing.

Walsh, D. (2009). Childbirth embodiment: Problematic aspects of current understandings. *Sociology of Health and Illness*, 32(3), 486–501.

Walsh, D., Spiby, H., Grigg, C., Dodwell, M., McCourt, C., Culley, L., Bishop, S., Wilkinson, J., Coleby, D., Pacanowski, L., Thornton, J., & Byers, S. (2018). Mapping midwifery and obstetric units in England. *Midwifery*, 56, 9–16. doi: 10.1016/j.midw.2017.09.009

Wax, J. R., Lucas, F. L., Lamont, M., Pinette, M. G., Cartin, A., & Blackstone, J. (2010). Maternal and newborn outcomes in planned home birth vs planned hospital births: A meta-analysis. *American Journal of Obstetrics and Gynecology*, 203(3), 243.e1–243.e8. doi: 10.1016/j.ajog.2010.05.028

Wears, R. (2015). Standardisation and its discontents. *Cognition, Technology & Work*, 17(1), 89–94. doi: 10.1007/s10111-014-0299-6

Weisz, G., Cambrosio, A., Keating, P., Knaapen, L., Schlich, T., & Tournay, V. (2007). The emergence of clinical practice guidelines. *The Milbank Quarterly*, 85(4), 691–727. doi: 10.1111/j.1468-0009.2007.00505.x

WHO. (2016). *WHO Recommendations on Antenatal Care for a Positive Pregnancy Experience*. Geneva: WHO. https://apps.who.int/iris/bitstream/handle/10665/250796/9789241549912-eng.pdf?sequence=1

Wieringa, S. (2017). Has evidence-based medicine ever been modern? A Latour-inspired understanding of a changing EBM. *Journal of Evaluation in Clinical Practice* 23(5), 964–970. doi: 10.1111/jep.12752

Yau, C. W. H., Leigh, B., Liberati, E., Punch, D., Dixon-Woods, M., & Draycott, T. (2020). Clinical negligence costs: Taking action to safeguard NHS sustainability. *BMJ*, 368, m552. doi: 10.1136/bmj.m552

3

COUNTER DISCOURSES

Resistance in action

Previous chapters have determined midwives are ideally placed to deliver woman-centred care that promotes and optimises women's normal physiological processes across the childbearing continuum – 'full-scope midwifery'. Most UK midwives are employed by the NHS – a large-scale institution. However, employed midwives are located within a conflicted position; a defined and regulated professional role, with legal obligations to fulfil their full scope of practice, yet, employee expectations do not always align with these professional obligations, creating tension. 'Guideline-centred' care, a distillation of medical hegemonic birth practices, explored in the previous chapter, is a cause of such tension and conflict, which centre on, and are heightened by institutionalised birth. Although community midwives may have greater freedom due to less surveillance: – hospital guidelines, and guideline-centred cultures, will govern practice across the work settings and influence all employed maternity professionals. Building on these arguments, this chapter will first centre on birthing women and people's voices contextualising their choices, and the midwifery care delivered within the sociocultural 'good' mothering discourse. Second, a discussion of the variations between midwives' beliefs, attitudes and philosophies will be presented; midwives are not a homogeneous group of professionals and intra-differences influence whether birth choices are supported. From exploring these differences, a journey through the first phase of research findings will illuminate how NHS midwives, supportive of alternative physiological birth choices, delivered this care.

Cultural tensions: The 'good' mother

Studies have explored women's experiences of alternative birth choices including freebirthing, an active decision to give birth with no professional present

DOI: 10.4324/9781003265443-3

(Greenfield et al., 2021; McKenzie & Montgomery, 2021); 'high-risk' home-births (Hollander et al., 2018); vaginal birth after caesarean (VBAC) at home or in a birth pool (Townsend et al., 2022).[1] Several systematic reviews have captured motivations for these choices (Feeley et al., 2015; Holten & de Miranda, 2016; Madeley et al., 2022). These include previous unsatisfactory or negative/traumatic birth experiences; seeking to retain control over the birthing experience; philosophies aligned with birth as a spiritual or religious event or where a belief safe birth is an undisturbed birth, therefore, without interference by health professionals. These decisions, like any pregnancy and birthing choices, sit within the wider sociocultural mothering discourses whereby women are subjected to established implicit and explicit societal expectations of 'good mothering' (Blaylock et al., 2022; Goodwin & Huppatz, 2010). While attitudes and norms may shift around what constitutes 'good' mothering, it often centres a feto-centric perspective (Oaks, 2000). As alternative physiological birthing choices tend to sit outside established cultural norms and mainstream ideas of birthing practices, birthing women and people may experience greater scrutiny, judgement or stigma for their choices (Feeley & Thomson, 2016; McMahon & Ashworth, 2020). Such scrutiny may come from maternity professionals, but also family members, friends and even the wider public (Blaylock et al., 2022; Roberts & Walsh, 2018). Together, the 'good' mother discourse and the wider discourses explored in Chapter 2 perpetuate and reinforce each other, therefore, understanding fetocentrism is crucial to situating these birth choices and the complexities, challenges and tensions arising within this space.

The introduction of the ultrasound scan in the 1970s meant for the first time doctors were able to 'see' the fetus and created a shift from viewing the mother-baby dyad as one to a two-person model; a newly discovered 'second patient' (Doyal, 1979) creating a space for increased medical dominance over childbearing (Cahill, 2000; Lyerly et al., 2008). Whilst women appear to have broadly embraced such technology (Garcia et al., 2002), some argue that the consequences have facilitated women's alienation from embodied knowledge of their pregnancies to reliance upon experts (Mitchell, 2001; Young, 2001). Moreover, the visibility of the fetus has created a cultural discourse in which women are viewed as 'containers' or 'vessels' or as Mitchell (2001) argues pregnant women have become 'living fetal monitors'. This can be viewed as women being a means to an end i.e., producers of a healthy live baby (Parry, 2008).

Cultural expectations of the 'production' of a healthy baby appear to have reduced societal tolerance for anything less than perfect (Healy et al., 2016; Surtees, 2010). Aligned with strong discourses regarding risk aversion and what Bisits (2016) calls the 'risk information explosion', pregnancy and birth became viewed as a particularly dangerous and risky time – despite evidence that pregnancy and childbirth have never been safer (Scamell & Alaszewski, 2012). Coxon et al. (2014) also suggested the contemporary parenting discourses influenced by popular media and culture emphasise the role of parents in becoming personal 'risk managers' in relation to birth, feeding and beyond. Such discourses place pressure and potential blame on individuals (in the event of poor or adverse outcomes) which ignore the structural factors[2] at play (Healy et al., 2016). These discourses can marginalise women's experiences, where the emphasis on fetal safety is prioritised over the mother's wellbeing (Mitchell, 2001; Parry, 2008). Dahlen & Homer (2013) refers to philosophical differences between notions of 'childbirth' and 'motherbirth'. The former relates to the perspective that a good mother prioritises the baby and takes no risks; the latter considers giving birth matters to a woman, so mother and baby have equal priority. Some feminist critics would suggest 'childbirth' philosophical frameworks dominate the discourse where women are vulnerable to strong social pressure to conform to being a 'good mother' (Cahill, 2000; Kitzinger, 2005).

Social pressure and fear narratives have coalesced with good mothering narratives to create a method of societal control over women (Cahill, 2000; Kitzinger, 2005; Newnham, 2014). The good mother is sacrificial, forgoes her needs for her children, and in the case of pregnancy forgoes her needs for the unborn; the good mother listens and acts upon medical advice, entrusts her pregnancy, birth, and baby to medical professionals in lieu of her own instincts (Bryant et al., 2007; Mitchell, 2001; Newnham, 2014). Acts of 'deviance' are equated with a 'bad mother' (Harvey et al., 2015; Maher & Saugeres, 2007; Miller, 2012). As the fetus became more visible via biotechnology, its status elevated, the good versus bad mother narratives became further entrenched and relates to reproductive rights restrictions. For example, restricted access to abortion services (Ginsberg & Shulman, 2021) increased surveillance via medics and social services such as when declining maternity care (Plested & Kirkham, 2016) and moralistic opposition to women's choices (Shallow, 2013; Viisainen, 2000). Therefore, these issues and discourses give rise to birth choices 'outside of the guidelines' as deviant practices.

Ethical tensions for, and between midwives

Within the context of complex mothering and maternity care discourses, midwives can be viewed as mediators, arbitrators and/or gatekeepers of women's choices. This role can be facilitative (Nicholls et al., 2016) or obstructive (Plested & Kirkham, 2016) dependent in part, on the tensions outlined in Chapter 2, and in part on differing midwives' philosophies. Notwithstanding the known tensions in midwifery practice, midwives have different belief systems and values and are not a homogenous group of professionals. Despite the unique, specific role and definition of a midwife (International Confederation of Midwives, 2017), how midwives are aligned can influence their attitude and willingness to facilitate alternative physiological birth choices (Feeley et al., 2019). Researchers have conceptualised these different alignments broadly as two extremes. One is based on a 'woman-centred' philosophy, where the holistic needs of the woman guide the care provided and autonomous decision-making is actively supported (Carolan & Hodnett, 2007; Hunter, 2004). This is opposed to a task-oriented approach, a 'guideline-centred' or 'with-institution' philosophy, where the needs of the organisation are prioritised over individual women (Crozier et al., 2007; Hunter, 2004).[3]

Furthermore, some midwives are aligned with a medical-technocratic perspective (Cooper, 2011) and/or a paternalistic approach to caregiving whereby women's autonomy is not central to belief and value systems (Thompson, 2005; Thompson, A., 2013). Viewed within an ethical lens, those not aligned with women's bodily autonomy and prioritise the needs of an institution, or hold a medical paternalistic, fetocentric philosophy, can negatively influence birthing women and people's access to, and experience of care (Newnham & Kirkham, 2019). Micro and macro restrictions to full bodily autonomy can occur, rendering commitments to maternal autonomy as (often, not always) rhetorical. Newnham & Kirkham (2019) impugned woman-centred rhetoric asserting it hides numerous unethical practices – persuasion, coercion, threats and withdrawal of care for those seeking care not conforming to medical-institutional norms.

Midwives with a woman-centred philosophy, but work within the confines of inflexible institutional norms, report significant challenges facilitating women's autonomy (Cobell, 2015). A lack of support, professional barriers and ongoing tensions among colleagues were cited as challenges when supporting alternative physiological births (Cobell, 2015; Hunter, 2004) – mirroring longstanding obstacles midwives have reported when delivering care that optimises physiological birth experiences (Ball et al., 2003). Previous research found midwives 'doing good by stealth' whereby they appease employee expectations with subtle lies to maintain an optimal physiological birth environment for the women (Kirkham, 1999). Other studies have reported active resistance against hegemonic birth practices (O'Connell & Downe, 2009; Reed, 2013), however, midwives have reported being reprimanded or even bullied (Edwards et al., 2011; Leap, 1997). Therefore, institutionally endorsed unethical practices, and a lack of commitment to maternal autonomy, can put midwives with a woman-centred philosophy in a morally distressing situation.[4] However, the rest of this chapter focuses on how the study participants specifically delivered alternative physiological birth care, adding to the research and counter-discourse. Subsequent chapters will share the experiences and impact of doing so, including both the positive and negative to add further contextual insights.

Resisting the status quo

Having discerned differing midwifery philosophies and the importance of recognising these differences, we return to the midwives in this study introduced in Chapter 1. To meet the aims of the research, the midwives recruited were those with a 'with-woman philosophy' – they willingly and proactively supported women's alternative physiological birth choices and it was a regular part of their practice.[5] Accordingly, the participants can be viewed as those resisting the status quo and having strong motivations to share their stories. For some, it was the first time their midwifery practice had been a focus of research attention, for others, they wanted to share extraordinary stories and for some, participating was an explicit act of 'resistance':

> I chose to share this story as an antidote to anger and resentment. I became a midwife because I wanted to protect and enhance women's health and their rights. It feels more and more that I am ensnared in a mad conspiracy which licenses obstetric butchery.
>
> *[Beatrice]*

The alternative physiological birth choices ranged from a 'nudge' outside of guidelines to a 'giant leap', with significant levels of complexity (see Appendix 2 for the range of birth decisions the participants were involved with). The choices included women who had healthy and uncomplicated pregnancies declining certain aspects of care (e.g., a postdate induction) and those with complicated pregnancies, with either obstetric or pre-existing health issues who wanted midwifery-led care (e.g., declining continuous electronic monitoring during vaginal birth after caesarean) and/or midwifery-led birth settings (home or birth centres). Between the 45 midwives, they provided hundreds of examples, likely capturing most possibilities. Although, what constitutes 'out of guidelines' for one midwife may not have been the same for another, as guidelines between different organisations vary. For example, at one institution supporting women with raised body mass index (BMI) in the pool was 'within' guidelines but elsewhere 'outside'. While in the UK the National Institute for Health and Care Excellence (NICE) generates guidelines to inform the national conversation, organisations are not required to follow them, thus variations exist.

The rest of this chapter follows the study findings to explore the actions and processes of how the midwives delivered alternative physiological birth care. These findings have been further developed since the PhD submission and subsequent journal publication (Feeley et al., 2020). Largely influenced by new thinking, reading and writing such as Newnham & Kirkham's (2019) argument for a care ethics approach in midwifery care, the original themes have been reconstructed to reflect these influences. Starting with how the midwives enacted supported decision-making (a core component of ethical care), their processes of facilitation are explored – 'responsive midwifery', 'safety constructed through relationships', 'tools not rules' and 'ethical competence'. Lucy, a study participant, summarises the sentiment of these overall research findings:

> As midwives working within the NHS, there are always going to be challenges, in every aspect of our role. But we are able to support women's choices, we may feel bound by guidelines but women are not. The outcome of not following best practice or Trust recommendations is not always going to be perfect, and we may perceive this as being dangerous or unnecessary, but it's not our choice to make. We must ensure that the

woman is fully informed, and provide woman-centred care, choice and advocation.

[Lucy]

Responsive midwifery

Where Chapters 1 and 2 highlighted barriers for those seeking alternative physiological births through protective steering, persuasion and coercive practices, here, we explore different responses. The birthing women and people presented their needs for decision-making to the midwives in a variety of ways; asserting a predetermined decision without any midwifery input required or wanted, uncertainty about options requiring help, information giving and support and for some, unawareness of options available to them. The following explores how the study participants responded and adapted to these individual needs demonstrating authentic 'supported decision-making', and enacting the ethical principles of respectful, dignified care (Kloester et al., 2022). Affirming, not resisting women's definitive decisions, collaborating with information giving and ensuring accessible information was provided to all women represented three proactive ways to support birthing women and people's different needs. Crucially, these findings demonstrate supported decision-making as an ongoing process and not (typically) a one-off conversation, nor can it be reduced to a tick box. Thus, it requires flexibility, responsiveness and required high levels of knowledge and skill. Furthermore, these three ways of achieving supported decision-making are not mutually exclusive, nor an either/or. Rather, they are multiple approaches to the same end, meeting the needs of those receiving care.

Some participants cared for women with clear birthing decisions who did not require input or information from any maternity professionals or the study participants. In these situations, the women asserted their decision and delineated their boundaries for the care they would or would not accept, including opting out of maternity care altogether should the midwives not support them. For example, Jenna cared for someone wanting a breech homebirth, and was prepared to freebirth should the service not support her decision. Jenna's response was pragmatic, preferring to facilitate the decision on the grounds of woman-centredness and safety, putting in place numerous measures designed to support the community midwives (with no experience of breech birth) so they could support the woman's decision.[6] Such decisions could be seen as threatening for professionals who might feel their professional autonomy or even their employment status was at risk following the woman's lead rather than employer expectations, and if they felt the decision was very risky (Feeley et al., 2019). However, the midwives in this study coped with these pressures, taking the longer-term view that women had reasons for their decisions. Perceived as safer than the alternative, affirming and proactively supporting women's decisions, was viewed as essential for women's engagement with services (Tomaselli et al., 2020). Exemplified by Maria, called to a homebirth 'just in case' where the woman declined all midwifery care or input but wanted Maria to be in the next room. In this situation, Maria demonstrated both willingness and confidence to meet her needs:

> … When I got to her flat a doula was present and the woman was mobilising and looked to be in established labour. She declined any baseline observations and told me she didn't want me to listen in to the baby at all, she said she'd called me just in case I was needed …
>
> *[Maria]*

In other situations, women were seeking varying levels of support, information and guidance to inform their decision-making. In these situations, the midwives' role was influential through the provision of information and navigating the maternity system to actualise the women's wishes – 'collaborative decision-making' occurred. Collaboration saw midwives as responsive to the requests of women in their care, sharing their resources (such as information or knowledge) to facilitate and empower women to achieve their preferences. This approach is highly reflective of an equitable, partnership model of practice and aligns with the kinds of models of informed decision-making in the broader health care literature (Begley et al., 2019; Kloester et al., 2022). For example, Sam was caring for a woman with epilepsy seeking a homebirth. Sam demonstrated a collaborative working relationship where her role was to actively seek evidence-based information, develop a care plan and deliver care based on the woman's preferences:

> Yea, I was working as a community midwife, and uhm, she had a uhm a disappointing birth experience with her first baby … She said 'you know I'd really like a homebirth, what would be me options?' I said 'well, leave it with me, I'll go away and have a look at what the evidence says but at the end of the day so as long as you are aware of the pros and cons and the fact that you have got epilepsy, it's your choice.'
>
> *[Sam]*

Different again were midwives who 'widened women's choices'. Rather than being directed by women's definitive decision-making or responding to their voiced preferences, a different way of enacting supported decision-making was reported. By avoiding assumptions such as prior knowledge of birth options and/or 'risk status', class, age, education, ethnicity, etc., extensive information was provided to all women in their care. The participants wanted to widen women's knowledge and access to different care options; therefore, the conversations were midwife-led but woman-driven. A key example was Kelly,[7] caring for someone with their fifth baby. Since the risks of labour are believed to increase after the fifth baby, many guidelines advise against homebirth in this situation. However, the woman had experienced very fast labour and birth for her most recent baby, almost not arriving at the hospital in time.[8] Kelly, therefore, suggested a homebirth, with due precautions – an option the woman had not known was available to her. Once the seed was sown, the woman went on to have several successful homebirths. Kelly believed giving full information about what is possible, to all women, without assumptions,[9] was ethically the right thing to do:

> … It's offering, it's giving everybody the whole range of choices. Not say-ing to her 'no you can't have your baby at home because you are high risk', it's going 'these are your choices, you know, what do you want to do? How do you want to take this?'

> [Kelly]

Echoing Kelly's ethos of care, others who reported widening women's choices held a strong ethos of ensuring women were provided with full information to make informed decisions. Like Kelly, other midwives observed that when women were given a wide range of options, their decisions *very rarely correspond exactly to the guidelines*, insinuating the information provided (or not) signifi-cantly influences decision-making. For example, Kerry caring for someone with a blood-borne virus seeking midwifery-led care, the woman originally requested the 'home from home' room at the obstetric unit. However, through a meaning-ful discussion with the Consultant Midwife, it created the space for the woman to request (and have) a homebirth. Therefore, extending the 'collaborative' partnership model, the midwives used their power to proactively open (widen) options otherwise unknown to the women in their care (Begley et al., 2019; Kloester et al., 2022).

Safety reconstructed through relationships

As discussed in Chapter 2, notions of 'safety' in maternity care have become reduced to hyperfocus on physical outcomes during the acute birth phase of the childbearing continuum, which can be biased towards a medicalised, interven-tionist approach. Therefore, concepts of 'safety' within the current hegemonic paradigm are unreliable and can be seen as devices to encourage conformity (Blaylock et al., 2022). To challenge this, safety needs to be reconstructed within a broader view and viewed holistically to encompass biological, psychological, social, spiritual and cultural elements[10] (Esegbona-Adeigbe, 2020; Olza et al., 2018). Viewing birthing women and people's decisions through a holistic safety lens offers a deeper understanding of their choices. While guidelines have been extensively critiqued, there are situations where decisions made are counter to strong evidence for physical wellbeing and safety. However, physical safety is not the only concern for many individuals and wider concerns (emotional, cultural, etc.) can be as, or more important, or weigh more heavily in decision-making (Madeley et al., 2022), thus requiring maternity professionals to enact a holistic approach.

A humanised approach to maternity care is a holistic approach, requiring maternity professionals to ascertain individual perceptions of safety of those in their care. What constitutes a significant risk for one person may be perceived as minor for someone else.[11] Ascertaining individuals' perceptions, values and 'material risks' to guide personalised care plans and delivery requires meaningful two-way conversations (Birthrights, 2020; Lokugamage & Pathberiya, 2017). While challenging within busy environments where significant time constraints occur, such conversations are the cornerstone of ethical practice, respectful, dignified and lawful care (Morton & Simkin, 2019). Ascertaining what is important with openness and honesty requires the cultivation of trusting relationships (Brown et al., 2011). In this context, relational care can be seen as a hallmark of safety in its broadest sense (Sandall et al., 2016). Unique to my study was how midwives articulated and 'unpacked' relational care, and how trusting relationships were achieved – whereby safety was reconstructed through relational care with understanding, support, trust and trustworthiness as key pillars of safe care.

'Listening to understand' was the first building block for the mother-midwife relationship reported by the midwives. Through listening, allowing time and space for women to open up, the midwives sought to understand the woman's perspective, her story and ethos around birth. As an important activity to build the foundations of trusting relationships, the midwives reported the women revealing many upsetting accounts of previous birth trauma and negative experiences of care. Such experiences were drivers of the women's alternative physiological birth choices, often with significant complexity. For example, Trish was caring for a woman with multiple medical complexities who wanted a twin home waterbirth. While the community midwives were alarmed at such a decision, Trish found through careful listening, the woman revealed the extent and impact of her previous traumatic hospital birth experience. To reclaim control was through homebirth. Taking the time to understand the woman's position Trish asked what her birthing 'non-negotiables' were:

> … The things that were non-negotiable though were not to do with clinical care. She wanted everyone who came in her room to introduce themselves, no one to touch her without asking permission and all changes to the plan to be explained to her first …

This finding was extremely important, Trish got to the heart of what constituted safety for this woman, less about birthplace and even midwifery-led care, but an issue of dignity and respect in the birth room (Morton & Simkin, 2019) – emotional safety. As it turned out, over time and in their ongoing relationship the woman did decide to have a hospital birth (with a very successful outcome). Where a hospital birth may have been the safer physical option, had this woman's emotional safety needs not been met first, it may have deterred engagement with maternity professionals. Where women do not feel supported, and/or lack trust in their caregivers, they are increasingly opting out of maternity care altogether

(Greenfield et al., 2021; McKenzie & Montgomery, 2021). For midwives who may be nervous in this situation, Trish's actions (and others in the study) highlight that through understanding the woman, what appears to be a seemingly radical (and perhaps alarming) complex birth decision becomes simpler and less alarming. Such is the power of relationships.

Proactively conveying support for women's birthing choices was integral to the midwives' ethical and philosophical approach. Stemming from a place of authenticity, the midwives wanted to be supportive, a core value underpinning their care and worked hard to express their support. This entailed a particular 'attitude' – a personal policy of not saying no. Doing this early on, when first meeting women, was reported as a way of breaking down potential barriers, disarming women who may have expected a 'battle'. Although it must be emphasised this was a genuine approach, with strong desires to support birthing women or people, and not a manipulative tactic to 'get women on side'. Such an attitude was based on a solutions-focused mindset, positive psychology, and the valuing of women's autonomous decision-making. Coupled with competence and confidence in their skillsets, the midwives were mostly unphased[12] by the range of birthing decisions presented:

> You have to go with what people want (laughs), you've got to pick your battles and fights and you will get more out of people if you say 'yes I'll support you in that but here you are, here are the risks', rather than saying 'no you can't, that doesn't really help anybody does it?
>
> *[Jane]*

Through this, midwives were forming and strengthening relationships, attempting to harness feelings of trust and psychological safety. However, their attitude did not mean a blasé approach, nor did it mean no further action, planning or discussions took place (discussed in later sections). However, it did mean starting from a baseline of support whereby conveying this was perceived as crucial to building trust, ensuring women's decision-making was informed, rather than reactionary to a lack of support. Therefore, supporting alternative physiological birth choices *is* safe care:

> … Being told 'you can't', 'I won't allow' 'no' can often create a communication problem that may encourage decisions based on fear of not being supported rather than a true assessment of risks and benefits.
>
> *[Jenny]*

Tools not rules

Where the overuse and overreliance on guidelines have pitfalls, and issues arise with the misapplication of evidence-based medicine as highlighted in Chapter 2, this section explores effective use, aligned with woman-centred care. Arguably, the midwives in this study were operationalising *evidence-informed* practice honouring the intention of the evidence-based medicine principles (Sackett, 1997). Evidence-informed practice (EIP) reinforces the centrality of patient (woman) needs, to which the professional combine what is known (current and up-to-date evidence) with clinical expertise offering recommendations *and* alternatives to create the space for authentic informed decision-making (Kumah et al., 2019). In this way, guidelines and evidence were used in conjunction with clinical expertise as *tools, not rules* to support women's alternative physiological birth choices – the essence of a relational model of care (Newnham & Kirkham, 2019). Through a proactive commitment to EIP based on current up-to-date evidence that centred on the needs of women, the participants reclaimed responsibility for their practice (Tronto, 1993) resisting a guideline, routine-centred approach to care:

> …usually at that point, cos they usually say quite early on in the pregnancy, I would say 'right well, you need me to have a look at the evidence, the up to date evidence to find out what the actual risks are for you individually, and then we will have a look at that together and have a discussion about whether you would still feel like you want to carry on with that birth, you know, after we've looked at the risks together really.
>
> *[Anna]*

Having extensive knowledge of their institutional guidelines was central to the midwives' ability to resist. Knowledge of what was deemed 'out of guidelines' coupled with cultural knowledge of what was locally acceptable or not was paramount in navigating the system in support of the women's choices. Alongside this, the midwives took a proactive stance of seeking out, accessing and assessing information from wider sources. Such activities underpin both evidence-informed practice (Kumah et al., 2019) and their professional obligations (NMC, 2018). The midwives reported extensive reading [around the specific clinical situation], joining research or professional online groups to keep abreast of new research, accessing national guidelines such as NICE/RCOG, liaising with medical professionals, seeking out other hospital guidelines and accessing primary research papers. Where there was little or no evidence to inform clinical practice, the midwives drew up knowledge from basic sciences, and clinical expertise (their own and that of others) to apply such knowledge to unique and individual situations.

Alex caring for someone with Group B Strep requesting a waterbirth at the birth centre was aware the local guidelines restricted access to both (birthing pool and birth centre). Having initially tried to advocate to her line manager, Alex was told firmly, '*no*' the woman was '*not allowed*' to attend the birth centre. However, Alex formally gathered information together, the latest research, and evidence and obtained guidelines from other organisations without these restrictions. The collated information was used successfully to advocate for the woman's birth choice, who went on to have a *'lovely waterbirth'* with Alex in attendance. In this example, Alex resisted the dominant culture aligned with the woman's preferences and through responsive midwifery, using wider evidence and external guidelines as tools to facilitate this birth choice

> …I wanted to facilitate that [her birth choice] the best way I can really. But I think that comes from, from educating yourself as well you know. I think some people would say 'that is just the way it is'. But I think you have to know your stuff to know actually that there is no reason Group B Strep means that a lady should have to go onto an obstetric unit.[13]
>
> *[Alex]*

Care plans, written by midwives, but based on the woman's decisions, were a tool commonly used by the midwives during the antenatal period. Care plans were a documented reflection of discussions including the risks, benefits, and alternatives, as well as an individualised risk assessment.[14] For some midwives, the care planning documentation was informal and the responsibility of the primary midwife. For others, there were formalised procedures in place including proformas or referrals to senior midwives (e.g., Consultant Midwives) and/or obstetricians who then wrote the care plan. Mostly, care planning documentation was viewed favourably for a multitude of reasons: as a tool to support women's decision-making, as a demonstration of commitment to the birthing choice, to reduce repetitive conversations with other professionals, to minimise the anxiety of other professionals, and a tool for advocacy in situations where women would be cared by other midwives during labour:

> … Ok, so it tends to be like women declining postdates induction or anyone who wants something outside of the guidance, it's probably better to have a plan I'd say even if it's something small to ensure that what they want will be honoured, I think it's easier for them to go into a situation with a doctor or a midwife and all this is going on and all of a sudden they feel like they don't have a voice anymore and they can't say what they want or need …
>
> *[Lucy]*

Moreover, for some, care plans *'contributed to the institutions ability to provide vicarious liability when caring for women outside of the conventional NHS menu'*. As such, care plans were viewed as multi-functional, serving the needs of the organisation, health professionals and women. The care plans appear to represent a means of legitimising women's decision-making and a mechanism for caregiving midwives that signalled institutional support for providing such care. Conversely, data from Katie highlighted care plans used in coercive ways. She reported management insisted a woman sign a care plan, pre-consenting to procedures for a home twin birth and with the inference of a disclaimer. All of these are fundamentally against the principles of consent legislation in the UK and should not have been carried out (Birthrights, 2020). Therefore, while in this study care plans mostly served positive purposes, negative unintended uses and consequences must be considered. Further research is required to explore care plans from wider perspectives including from birthing women and people in receipt of them.

Ethical competence

Where research shows many women want a physiological birth, as explored in Chapter 1, they are also prepared to 'go with the flow' in the event of unplanned events or emergencies (Downe et al., 2018). However, women in these studies do expect maternity providers to have the skills to facilitate physiological labour and birth competently and safely (Downe et al., 2018), arguably an ethical imperative for maternity professionals to provide care adequately and competently (Tronto, 1993). Extending this, birthing women and people likely expect the health systems to be set up to facilitate physiological births but as we have seen in Chapter 2, the declining physiological birth rates and disparities between birthplace settings demonstrate otherwise. Again, arguably, an ethical imperative for health systems to provide enabling, evidence-based environments. The midwives in this study navigated and overcame organisational complexities favouring hegemonic medicalised birth practices, through ethical competence across a broad range of skills. Related to intrapartum care, these skills included appropriate knowledge and preparedness for potential and/or emerging pathology and competence to offer and/or deliver (if consented to) judicious interventions as required. Thus, avoiding a blasé approach or as Dahlen (2010) suggested a 'sentimental [normal] birth ideology' which may ignore existing or emerging clinical situations that require both recognition (knowledge) and action (transfer, help-seeking, procedures or interventions).

Fundamentally, the study participants in this study illuminated how to create the necessary conditions to improve women's likelihood of experiencing their wanted physiological birth but with readiness and preparedness for the unpredictability of childbirth. A strength of care planning during pregnancy was to incorporate contingency and mitigation planning within a low-stress antenatal environment, so women can consider all possibilities and remain the decision-maker during the intrapartum period (a potentially stressful situation). Additionally, preparedness may have included specific activities designed to support midwife caregivers including educational activities, simulated practice (skills and drills for emergencies) and setting up specific on-call teams. This could be summed up as 'planning for the worst, anticipating the best' outcome:

> I think I am quite an organised person and knowing that we'd been through every scenario very clearly helped me, knowing we had covered all bases

and planning uhm I always set myself up for the worst-case scenario, which
some people don't really agree with (laughs) …

[Lucy supporting a woman having a home VBAC]

Similarly, Stella described a situation where despite meticulous planning for a
breech birth at the alongside birth centre, the woman went into spontaneous labour
and progressed rapidly at home leaving little time for transfer. A quick decision to
remain at home was made in collaboration with the woman and her partner. This
situation benefitted from extensive collaborative antenatal planning, whereby all
birthplace options were discussed, considered and planned for. Therefore, the situation was less surprising or challenging as previous care plans which could be
quickly operationalised e.g., calling the second midwife, informing the supervisor
on call and having an ambulance on standby. The outcome resulted in a safe home
breech birth, requiring some skilled midwifery input to facilitate the birth:

> I did a gentle Mauriceau-Cronk manoeuvre to free the crown, and Mai-
> sie landed Felix on the floor beautifully. He was shocked and a little flat,
> needing some resus (as we expected), but we did this on the floor, without
> cutting the cord – Apgar's of 5 & 9. The placenta came quickly, and she
> was on the sofa half an hour after the birth, breastfeeding with an intact
> perineum, wearing the hugest smile. Hugs and tea all round, and certain
> sense of relief. I do remember the second midwife having to take up the
> mantle a little after the placenta came away, as I was wandering around in
> a sort of ecstatic daze. I couldn't believe that, after all the pressure, it had
> happened some quickly, and so textbook…. the nicest reward for me was
> on being invited to the Felix's first birthday party – there was a note on my
> placemat, from Felix, saying: "Thanks for having the balls to stand by me
> when everyone else wouldn't".[15]

Crucially, ethical competence is also related to recognising the parameters and
limitations of their midwifery expertise. In some situations, as necessary, the
midwives sought collaborative input from the multi-disciplinary team to support safe care planning for women with health conditions, such as epilepsy,
cardiac conditions, or diabetes, or for babies anticipated to have post-birth complications. Some midwives reported challenging encounters with wider teams
(explored further in Chapter 4), but others reported good constructive working
relationships. For example, Kerry (mentioned earlier) was supporting a woman
with a blood-borne virus having a homebirth and sought the input of the wider
team – obstetricians, neonatologists, and specialist doctors. Kerry delineated her
area of expertise while remaining open to constructive input from the medics,
another way to demonstrate ethical competence:

> I think it is always the same thing, just the communication being really
> honest and listening to them [medics] as well and making sure, cos I'm not

an expert in the follow-up care [post birth antiretrovirals] … but reassuring them that I am an expert in normal birth, our homebirth rate was 35% so I was very confident that if things weren't going to happen we would transfer in and definitely listening to them, and knowing I wasn't that expert because although we were happy to support her but there may have been specialist genuine reasons why we'd have to think of alternatives and stuff.

[Kerry]

What has been achieved, what is possible?

This chapter has journeyed through the accounts of NHS midwives who have supported a wide range of alternative physiological birth choices. Aligned and committed to a 'with-woman' philosophy, their accounts offer a counter-discourse to the prevailing dominance of routine-based, institutionalised, medicalised and technocratic birth practices. Their resistance to the dominant discourses provides insights and learning opportunities for other maternity professionals and those receiving maternity care who want something similar; for examining how things have been done, lessons can be applied elsewhere. Furthermore, the study participants' articulation of the different components of relational care, how this was enacted, achieved and its impact supported new conceptualisations and understandings of what this looks like in everyday practice. Moreover, the insights of how to use guidelines and evidence as tools, not rules, help to reclaim evidence-based practice to one that is evidence-*informed,* and aligned with the original intentions of EBM. Ethical competence highlighted the range of skills required to facilitate any birth, not least those outside of the guidelines, illustrating 'full-scope' midwifery in action. However, having only touched on their experiences within their workplace, the next chapter will offer a deep dive into the conflicts and challenges which affected some of the midwives in the study.

Notes

1 For further reading on the range of studies explored birthing women and people's alternative physiological birth choices see Chapter 1, endnote 14.
2 Structural factors include issues such as class, socio-economic status ethnicity etc. But also include the broad sociocultural-political drivers discussed in Chapter 2 such as medicalisation, institutionalisation, risk, litigation discourses etc.
3 For further insights around differing midwifery philosophies see my PhD Thesis (Feeley, 2019).
4 For many, these challenges are associated with high levels of stress, burn out, and is a leading cause of leaving the profession and explored further in later chapters. For further reading, see (Alexander & Bogossian, 2018; Ball et al., 2003; Curtis et al., 2006; Hunter et al., 2019; Robertson & Thomson, 2016).
5 While this was the aim and every effort was made during recruitment, during data collection, one participant shared some conflicting feelings around supporting alternative physiological birth choices, primarily around support structures within their workplaces and/or lack of experience, see (Feeley, 2019).

6 Jenna, as a Consultant Midwife was responsible for providing complex care plans for birth choices 'outside of guidelines'. Her role was to provide support both for women and the potential midwife caregivers across the maternity service. In this example, a breech homebirth, Jenna provided extensive insights regarding the multiple conversations and support packages put in place for the woman and staff. Honesty was paramount and. Jenna reported transparent conversations with the woman who wished to continue with homebirth planning despite a lack of experienced midwives (a significant safety issue), to which Jenna put in place numerous training sessions and wrote an extensive care plan categorically delineating the roles and responsibilities for each person within the care team including the woman, partner and doula. This care plan was developed and written collaboratively with the woman with ambulance cover arranged should an emergency during the second stage of labour arise. While Jenna raised concerned around the resource allocation and resource disparity across the population of women the organisation serves, Jenna maintained support for the woman's decision. The woman went on to have a successful home breech birth with midwifery care.
7 Kelly, a participant, coined the term 'widening women's choices'.
8 An unexpected birth before arrival (BBA) can be very distressing for families and ideally avoided (Vik et al., 2016).
9 In Kelly's wider narratives she explained that women in her caseload were not all educated white middle class women who she believed, tended to know options and assert their decisions. Kelly observed disparities in women from different backgrounds as less likely to be offered the full range of choices and/or discouraged from meaningful informed decision-making. Her practice sought to address these disparities.
10 This is particularly relevant as ideas of cultural safety become magnified, with racist discrimination repeatedly exposed across many high-income countries, campaigners, service users are rightfully demanding sensitively delivered culturally safe care (Birthrights, 2022a; Birthrights, 2022b; Esegbona-Adeigbe, 2020; Hartz et al., 2019).
11 Induction of labour for prolonged pregnancy is a typical example of where perceptions of safety/risk can be radically different. Where there is an increased risk of stillbirth >42 weeks (usually cited as 1 to 2:1000 for otherwise healthy women) (NICE, 2017) for some birthing women and people, this a serious risk and prefer induction to safeguard against a potential stillbirth. Conversely, for others, this is a small risk with the perceived risks of induction outweigh the potential protective effect of an induction.
12 A couple of the participants were less experienced than others in the study, and in their longer narratives, there were some clinical situations they felt less confident to manage – see (Feeley, 2019) for some insights around this.
13 The evidence for GBS screening and intrapartum management was (in 2017 when data was collected), and still is conflicting, with proponents on either side of the discussion. Currently, there is a large multi-centre RCT exploring GBS - see, https://www.gbs3trial.ac.uk/home.aspx. Moreover, regardless of the findings, birthing women and people still have the right to decline screening or prophylatic antibiotics.
14 Fully individualised risk assessments are challenging for those with multiple morbidities or complexities as much of the evidence available relates to single risk factors.
15 Pseudonyms were used throughout.

References

Alexander, C. R., & Bogossian, F. (2018). Midwives and clinical investigation: A review of the literature. *Women and Birth: Journal of the Australian College of Midwives*, 31(6), 442–452. doi: 10.1016/j.wombi.2018.02.003
Ball, L., Curtis, P., & Kirkham, M. (2003). *Why Do Midwives Leave? Talking to the Managers*. (No. 1). London: Royal College of Midwives.

Begley, K., Daly, D., Panda, S., & Begley, C. (2019). Shared decision-making in maternity care: Acknowledging and overcoming epistemic defeaters. *Journal of Evaluation in Clinical Practice*, 25(6), 1113–1120. doi: 10.1111/jep.13243

Birthrights. (2020). *Consenting to Treatment.* https://www.birthrights.org.uk/factsheets/consenting-to-treatment/

Birthrights. (2022a). *Inquiry on Racial Injustice in Maternity Care.* Terms of reference. https://www.birthrights.org.uk/campaigns-research/racial-injustice/

Birthrights. (2022b). *Systemic Racism, Not Broken Bodies: An Inquiry into Racial Injustice and Human Rights in UK Maternity Care.* https://www.birthrights.org.uk/wp-content/uploads/2022/05/Birthrights-inquiry-systemic-racism_exec-summary_May-22-web.pdf

Bisits, A. (2016). Risk in obstetrics: Perspectives and reflections. *Midwifery*, 38, 12–13. doi: 10.1016/j.midw.2016.05.010

Blaylock, R., Trickey, H., Sanders, J., & Murphy, C. (2022). WRISK voices: A mixed-methods study of women's experiences of pregnancy-related public health advice and risk messages in the UK. *Midwifery*, 113, 103433. doi: 10.1016/j.midw.2022.103433

Brown, P., Alaszewski, A., Swift, T., & Nordin, A. (2011). Actions speak louder than words: The embodiment of trust by healthcare professionals in gynae-oncology. *Sociology of Health & Illness*, 33(2), 280–295. doi: 10.1111/j.1467–9566.2010.01284.x

Bryant, J., Porter, M., Tracy, S., & Sullivan, E. (2007). Caesarean birth: Consumption, safety, order, and good mothering. *Social Science & Medicine* (1982), 65(6), 1192–1201. doi: 10.1016/j.socscimed.2007.05.025

Cahill, H. (2000). Male appropriation and medicalization of childbirth: An historical analysis. *Journal of Advanced Nursing*, 33(3), 334–342.

Carolan, M., & Hodnett, E. (2007). A 'with woman' philosophy: Examining the evidence, answering the questions. *Nursing Inquiry*, 14(2), 140–152. doi: 10.1111/j.1440–1800.2007.00360.x

Cobell, A. (2015). What are midwives' experiences of looking after women in labour outside of Trust guidelines? Master's Thesis: King's College London.

Cooper, T. (2011). Perceptions of the midwife's role: A feminist technoscience perspective. University of Central Lancashire. Doctoral Thesis: University of Central Lancashire.

Coxon, K., Sandall, J., & Fulop, N. (2014). To what extent are women free to choose where to give birth? How discourses of risk, blame and responsibility influence birthplace decisions. 16(1), 51–67. doi: 10.1080/13698575.2013.859231

Crozier, K., Sinclair, M., Kernohan, G., & Porter, S. (2007). The development of a theoretical model of midwifery competence in birth technology. *Evidence Based Midwifery*, 5(4); 119–121.

Curtis, P., Ball, L., & Kirkham, M. (2006). Why do midwives leave? (not) being the kind of midwife you want to be. *British Journal of Midwifery*, 14(1), 27–31.

Dahlen, H. (2010). Undone by fear? Deluded by trust? *Midwifery*, 26(2), 156–162. doi: 10.1016/j.midw.2009.11.008

Dahlen, H. G. & Homer, C. S. E. (2013). 'Motherbirth or childbirth'? A prospective analysis of vaginal birth after caesarean blogs. 29(2), 167–173. doi: 10.1016/j.midw.2011.11.007

Downe, S., Finlayson, K., Oladapo, O., Bonet, M., & Gülmezoglu, A. (2018). What matters to women during childbirth: A systematic qualitative review. 13(4). doi: 10.1371/journal.pone.0194906

Doyal, L. (1979). *The Political Economy of Health.* Pluto Press.

Edwards, N., Murphy-Lawless, J., Kirkham, M., & Davies, S. (2011). Attacks on midwives, attacks on women's choices. *Association for Improvements in the Maternity Services*, 23(3), 1–9.

Esegbona-Adeigbe, S. (2020). Cultural safety in midwifery practice – Protecting the cultural identity of the woman. *The Practising Midwife*, 23(11), 10–12.

Feeley, C. (2019). 'Practising outside of the box, whilst within the system': A feminist narrative inquiry of NHS midwives supporting and facilitating women's alternative physiological birthing choices. Doctoral Thesis: University of Central Lancashire.

Feeley, C., Burns, E., Adams, E., & Thomson, G. (2015). Why do some women choose to freebirth? A meta-thematic synthesis, part one. *Evidence Based Midwifery*, 13(1), 4–9.

Feeley, C., & Thomson, G. (2016). Tensions and conflicts in 'choice': Women's' experiences of freebirthing in the UK. *Midwifery*, 41, 16–21. doi: 10.1016/j.midw.2016.07.014

Feeley, C., Thomson, G., & Downe, S. (2019). Caring for women making unconventional birth choices: A meta-ethnography exploring the views, attitudes, and experiences of midwives. *Midwifery*, 72, 50–59. doi: 10.1016/j.midw.2019.02.009

Feeley, C., Thomson, G., & Downe, S. (2020). Understanding how midwives employed by the National Health Service facilitate women's alternative birthing choices: Findings from a feminist pragmatist study. *Plos One*, 15(11), e0242508. doi: 10.1371/journal.pone.0242508

Garcia, J., Bricker, L., Henderson, J., Martin, M., Mugford, M., Nielson, J., & Roberts, T. (2002). Women's views of pregnancy ultrasound: A systematic review. *Birth*, 29(4), 225–250.

Ginsberg, N. A., & Shulman, L. P. (2021). Life without Roe v Wade. *Contraception and Reproductive Medicine*, 610. doi: 1186/s40834-021-00149-6

Goodwin, S., & Huppatz, K. E. (2010). The good mother in theory and research: An overview. In S. Goodwin & K. Huppatz (Eds.), *The Good Mother: Contemporary Motherhoods in Australia* (pp. 1–24). Sydney University Press: Sydney.

Greenfield, M., Payne-Gifford, S., & McKenzie, G. (2021). Between a rock and a hard place: Considering "freebirth" during Covid-19. *Frontiers in Global Women's Health*, 2, 603744. doi: 010.3389/fgwh.2021.603744

Hartz, D. L., Blain, J., Caplice, S., Allende, T., Anderson, S., Hall, B., McGrath, L., Williams, K., Jarman, H., & Tracy, S. K. (2019). Evaluation of an Australian Aboriginal model of maternity care: The Malabar community midwifery link service. *Women & Birth*, 32(5), 427–436. https://search.ebscohost.com/login.aspx?direct=true&db=cin20&AN=138152052&site=ehost-live

Harvey, S., Schmied, V., Nicholls, D., & Dahlen, H. (2015). Hope amidst judgement: The meaning mothers accessing opioid treatment programmes ascribe to interactions with health services in the perinatal period. *Journal of Family Studies*, 21(3), 282–304. doi: 10.1080/13229400.2015.1110531

Healy, S., Humphreys, E., & Kennedy, C. (2016). Can maternity care move beyond risk? Implications for midwifery as a profession. *British Journal of Midwifery*, 24(3), 203–209. doi: 10.12968/bjom.2016.24.3.203

Hollander, M., Holten, L., Leusin, A., & van Dillen, J. (2018). Less or more? Maternal requests that go against medical advice. Online, 1–8. doi: 10.1016/j.wombi.2018.01.010

Holten, L., & de Miranda, E. (2016). Women's motivations for having unassisted childbirth or high-risk homebirth: An exploration of the literature on 'birthing outside the system'. *Midwifery*, 38, 55–62. doi: 10.1016/j.midw.2016.03.010

Hunter, B. (2004). Conflicting ideologies as a source of emotion work in midwifery. *Midwifery*, 20(3), 261–272.

Hunter, B., Fenwick, J., Sidebotham, M., & Henley, J. (2019). Midwives in the United Kingdom: Levels of burnout, depression, anxiety and stress and associated predictors. *Midwifery*, 79, 102526. doi: 7910.1016/j.midw.2019.08.008

International Confederation of Midwives. (2017). ICM definitions: Definition of the midwife. https://www.internationalmidwives.org/our-work/policy-and-practice/icm-definitions.html#:~:text=The%20midwife%20is%20recognised%20as, the%20newborn%20and%20the%20infant

Kirkham, M. (1999). The culture of midwifery in the NHS in England. *British Journal of Midwifery*, 30(3), 732–739.

Kitzinger, S. (2005). *The Politics of Birth*. Elsevier.

Kloester, J., Willey, S., Hall, H., & Brand, G. (2022). Midwives' experiences of facilitating informed decision-making – a narrative literature review. *Midwifery*, 109, 103322. doi: 10.1016/j.midw.2022.103322

Kumah, E. A., McSherry, R., Bettany-Saltikov, J., Hamilton, S., Hogg, J., Whittaker, V., & Schaik, P. V. (2019). PROTOCOL: Evidence-informed practice versus evidence-based practice educational interventions for improving knowledge, attitudes, understanding, and behavior toward the application of evidence into practice: A comprehensive systematic review of undergraduate students. *Campbell Systematic Reviews*, 15(1–2), e1015. doi: 10.1002/cl2.1015

Leap, N. (1997). Making sense of horizontal violence in midwifery. *British Journal of Midwifery*, 5(11), 689. doi: 10.12968/bjom.1997.5.11.689

Lokugamage, A. U., & Pathberiya, S. D. C. (2017). Human rights in childbirth, narratives and restorative justice: A review. *Reproductive Health*, 14(1), 17. doi: 10.1186/s12978-016-0264-3

Lyerly, A. D., Little, M. O., & Faden, R. R. (2008). A critique of the 'fetus as patient'. *The American Journal of Bioethics*, 8(7), 42–44. doi: 10.1080/15265160802331678

Madeley, A., Earle, S., & Boyle, S. (2022). What are the views, attitudes, perceptions and experiences of women who make non-normative choices along maternity care pathways? *Midwifery*, In Press.

Maher, J., & Saugeres, L. (2007). To be or not to be a mother?: Women negotiating cultural representations of mothering. *Journal of Sociology*, 43(1), 5–21. doi: 10.1177/1440783307073931

McKenzie, G., & Montgomery, E. (2021). Undisturbed physiological birth: Insights from women who freebirth in the United Kingdom. *Midwifery*, 101, 103042. doi: 10.1016/j.midw.2021.103042

McMahon, M., & Ashworth, E. (2020). *Social Care Referrals: Lifting the Lid*. https://www.all4maternity.com/social-care-referrals-lifting-the-lid/

Miller, A. (2012). On the margins of the periphery: Unassisted childbirth and the management of layered stigma. *Sociological Spectrum*, 32(5), 406–423. doi: 10.1080/02732173.2012.694795

Mitchell, M. (2001). *Baby's First Picture: Ultrasound and the Politics of Fetal Subjects*. University of Toronto Press.

Morton, C., & Simkin, P. (2019). Can respectful maternity care save and improve lives? *Birth*, 46(3), 391–395. doi: 10.1111/birt.12444

Newnham, E. (2014). Birth control: Power/knowledge in the politics of birth. *Health Sociology Review*, 23(3), 254–268. doi: 10.1080/14461242.2014.11081978

Newnham, E., & Kirkham, M. (2019). Beyond autonomy: Care ethics for midwifery and the humanization of birth. *Nursing Ethics*, 26(7–8), 2147–2157. 10.1177/0969733018819119

NICE. (2017). *Intrapartum Care for Healthy Women and Babies*. NICE. https://www. nice.org.uk/guidance/cg190/resources/intrapartum-care-for-healthy-women-and-babies-pdf-35109866447557

Nicholls, S., Hauck, Y. L., Bayes, S., & Butt, J. (2016). Exploring midwives' perception of confidence around facilitating water birth in Western Australia: A qualitative descriptive study. *Midwifery*, 33, 73–81. doi: 10.1016/j.midw.2015.10.010

NMC. (2018). *The Code Professional Standards of Practice and Behaviour for Nurses, Midwives and Nursing Associates*. London: Nursing and Midwifery Council. https://www.nmc. org.uk/globalassets/sitedocuments/nmc-publications/nmc-code.pdf

Oaks, L. (2000). Smoke-filled wombs and fragile fetuses: The social politics of fetal representation. *Signs*, 26(1), 63–108.

O'Connell, R., & Downe, S. (2009). A metasynthesis of midwives' experience of hospital practice in publicly funded settings: Compliance, resistance and authenticity. *Health: An Interdisciplinary Journal for the Social Study of Health, Illness and Medicine*, 13(6), 589–609.

Olza, I., Leahy-Warren, P., Benyamini, Y., Kazmierczak, M., Karlsdottir, S., Spyridou, A., Crespo-Mirasol, E., TakÃ¡cs, L., Hall, P., Murphy, M., Jonsdottir, S., Downe, S., & Nieuwenhuijze, M. (2018). Women's psychological experiences of physiological childbirth: A meta-synthesis. *BMJ Open*, 8(10). doi: 10.1136/bmjopen-2017–020347

Parry, D. (2008). We wanted a birth experience, not a medical experience: Exploring Canadian women's use of midwifery. *Health Care for Women International*, 29(8), 784–806. doi: 10.1080/07399330802269451

Plested, M., & Kirkham, M. (2016). Risk and fear in the lived experience of birth without a midwife. *Midwifery*, 38, 29–34. doi: 10.1016/j.midw.2016.02.009

Reed, R. (2013). Midwifery practice during birth: Rites of passage and rites of protection. Doctoral Thesis: University of Sunshine Coast.

Roberts, J., & Walsh, D. (2018). Babies come when they are ready: Women 's experiences of resisting the medicalisation of prolonged pregnancy. *Feminism & Psychology*, 29(1), 40–57. doi: 10.1177/0959353518799386

Robertson, J. H., & Thomson, A. M. (2016). An exploration of the effects of clinical negligence litigation on the practice of midwives in England: A phenomenological study. *Midwifery*, 33, 55–63. doi: 10.1016/j.midw.2015.10.005

Sackett, D. (1997). Evidence-based medicine. *Seminars in Perinatology*, 21(1), 3.

Sandall, J., Coxon, K., Mackingtosh, N., Rayment-Jones, H., Locock, L., & Page, L. (2016). Relationships: The Pathway to Safe, High-Quality Maternity Care Report from the Sheila Kitzinger Symposium at Green Templeton College October 2015. Oxford: King's College London. https://www.gtc.ox.ac.uk/images/stories/academic/ skp_report.pdf

Scamell, M., & Alaszewski, A. (2012). Fateful moments and the categorisation of risk: Midwifery practice and the ever-narrowing window of normality during childbirth. *Health, Risk & Society*, 14(2), 207–221. doi: 10.1080/13698575.2012.661041

Shallow, H. (2013). Deviant mothers and midwives: Supporting VBAC with women as real partners in decision making. *Essentially MIDIRS*, 4(1), 17–21.

Surtees, R. (2010). 'Everybody expects the perfect baby … and perfect labour … and so you have to protect yourself': Discourses of defence in midwifery practice in Aotearoa/ New Zealand. *Nursing Inquiry*, 17(1), 82–92. doi: 10.1111/j.1440–1800.2009.00464.x

Thompson, A. (2005). The emotional impact on mothers and midwives of conflict between workplace and personal/professional ethics. *Australian Midwifery Journal*, 18(3), 17–21.

Thompson, A. (2013). Midwives' experiences of caring for women whose requests are not within clinical policies and guidelines. *British Journal of Midwifery*, 21(8), 564–570. doi: 10.12968/bjom.2013.21.8.564

Tomaselli, G., Buttigieg, S. C., Rosano, A., Cassar, M., & Grima, G. (2020). Person-centered care from a relational ethics perspective for the delivery of high quality and safe healthcare: A scoping review. *Frontiers in Public Health*, 8, 44. doi: 10.3389/fpubh.2020.00044

Townsend, B., Fenwick, J., McInnes, R., & Sidebotham, M. (2022). Taking the reins: A grounded theory study of women's experiences of negotiating water immersion for labour and birth after a previous caesarean section. *Women and Birth*, In Press. doi: 10.1016/j.wombi.2022.07.171

Tronto, J. (1993). *Moral Boundaries: A Political Argument for an Ethic of Care*. Routledge.

Viisainen, K. (2000). The moral dangers of home birth: Parents' perceptions of risks in home birth in Finland. *Sociology of Health & Illness*, 22(6), 792–814. doi: 10.1111/1467–9566.00231

Vik, E. S., Haukeland, G. T., & Dahl, B. (2016). Women's experiences with giving birth before arrival. *Midwifery*, 42, 10–15. doi: 10.1016/j.midw.2016.09.012

Young, I. (2001). Pregnant embodiment. In D. Welton (Ed.), *Body and Flesh: A Philosophical Reader* (pp. 274–285). Blackwell Publishers.

4
MORAL COMPROMISE AND DISTRESS
Midwives' invisible wounds

Having explored how NHS midwives with a woman-centred philosophy and a proactive approach facilitate alternative physiological births, in this chapter, we will turn to their experiences. All NHS organisations reside under the same broad sociocultural landscapes described in Chapter 2. However, within this broader landscape, individual institutions have differing sociocultural-political norms giving rise to unique workplace cultures. The study participants were recruited from different organisations; therefore, varying workplace experiences were expected. However, this chapter and the next reveal an unexpected degree of polarisation across the accounts. Here, the focus is on the midwives who experienced challenging working environments. Captured as 'Stories of distress', we see how the sociocultural-political discourses of hegemonic birth practices and a 'guideline-centred' culture played out negatively affecting 19 of the study participants. While Chapter 3 highlighted the midwives' successes in supporting alternative physiological births, this was not always consistently possible or came at great cost. First, this chapter will explore the evidence of what midwives need to flourish within the workplace. Second, to situate the midwives' negative experiences, concepts of moral compromise and distress will be presented. The rest of the chapter illustrates the degrees of moral distress through emotion-stories of feeling torn, battle, reproach, recrimination and vilification.

Emotion stories: Moral distress and the workplace

As human beings, our rich internal landscape is mediated by our emotions and reactions to the interaction we have with the world we live in. How we make sense of ourselves, our lives and experiences is largely an emotional process developed through complex interacting layers of beliefs, attitudes, values, previous experiences, traumas, sociocultural influences, etc. As such, emotional reactions

DOI: 10.4324/9781003265443-4

illuminate both the obvious emotions (anger/joy) and the subtle (morose/contentment) to reveal ways in which meaning is created; and through storytelling, it can reveal that which is hidden. The second analysis examined the midwives' accounts through this lens of 'emotionality' (Kleres, 2011); the midwives in this research all had 'emotion-stories' expressing the everyday lived experience of delivering out of guideline care. For some, incongruent workplace environments confronted and violated their strongly-held values and for others, working within contexts of alignment, cultivated feelings of awe and wonder (see Chapter 5). Either way, the act(s) of delivering this care was not neutral, it was deeply personal and had long-lasting impacts. Moreover, the accounts highlighted the direct influence their workplace environment had on their experiences, the good and bad. Crucially, where the midwives worked, who they worked with, and the overall culture and politics of the organisation were highly influential in their stories and emotional sense-making.

Through numerous practice examples, 19 of the midwives in this study provided insights into the everyday frictions of delivering woman-centred care. Collectively, the accounts bring to life the recent recommendations from The King's Fund (2020). Their (independent) report, recognising the need to transform healthcare and culture, sought to identify what midwives need to deliver high-quality care (King's Fund, 2020). Acknowledging longstanding issues of consistent (persistent) workplace stressors, poor organisational cultures, working contexts and leadership as all have a detrimental impact on staffing recruitment, retention and wellbeing, the report developed recommendations to support the needs of midwives to ensure staff engagement, wellbeing and flourishing. The three core needs are autonomy – the need to have control over one's work life, and to be able to act consistently with one's values; belonging – the need to be connected to, cared for by, and be caring of colleagues, to feel valued, respected and supported; and contribution – the need to experience effectiveness in work and deliver valued outcomes (King's Fund, 2020). This chapter will demonstrate the experience and impact of not having these needs met, framed within notions of moral compromise, distress and injury (Litz & Kerig, 2019),[1] thus highlighting the trials and tribulations of the midwives' acts of resistance when supporting alternative physiological births.

Moral compromise or frustrations, distress and injury[2] encompass a continuum; from minor conflicts of one's morality with little long-term impact, all the way through to an irrecoverable injury (Litz & Kerig, 2019). Central to this continuum is where people are harmed by their own morally transgressive behaviour; the harm they may inflict through their own actions (or inactions) while violating their moral values (Litz & Kerig, 2019). This is different to ethical dilemmas where two options may have disadvantages yet be of equal ethical grounding or justification where the challenge is the decision-making. Conversely, the continuum of moral compromise to injury focuses on knowing the right thing to do, but not doing so (Jameton, 1984; Litz & Kerig, 2019). While definitions and clinical expressions of this continuum are currently in flux (due to the rapidly developing field of inquiry), this basic explanation can be considered within a healthcare delivery context. For example, Jameton (1984) captured moral distress as the negative psychological impact of complex ethical challenges in nursing, specifically where the nurse is morally constrained: 'moral distress occurs when one knows the right thing to do, but institutional constraints make it nearly impossible' (p. 6).

Jameton's (1984) early definition has been further developed by Fourie (2017) to consider 'moral constraint distress' (institutional constraints) and 'moral uncertainty distress' (not knowing what the morally right course of action is). The former is most relevant for the midwives in this chapter where some (explored below) experienced repeated exposure to moral constraint distress (Epstein & Hamric, 2009; Fourie, 2017). Repeated exposure leads to a cumulative effect, further compounded if/when health professionals' moral concerns have not been acknowledged (Epstein & Hamric, 2009). Epstein & Hamric (2009) found a lack of acknowledgement heightened health professionals' feelings of powerlessness and voicelessness creating a 'moral residue' – an amplification of moral distress. When concerns are repeatedly not heard or dismissed, distressing feelings may peak into a 'crescendo' leading to moral injury; whereby healthcare workers may become desensitised or morally numb, burned out and/or leave the profession (Epstein & Hamric, 2009). Therefore, the continuum of moral compromise to injury is vital in our understanding of the influence and impact when organisational values (culture and politics) intersect with those with differing values. Applied to midwifery, Foster et al., (2022) recently carried out a concept analysis to understand how moral distress can be best understood in midwifery practice. They developed a preliminary definition, of which moral constraint is most pertinent for the midwives in this study:

> a psychological suffering following clinical situations of moral uncertainty and/or constraint, which result in an experience of personal powerlessness where the midwife perceives an inability to preserve all competing moral commitments.
>
> *(Foster et al., 2022, p. 15)*

Stories of distress

Stories of feeling torn

In Chapter 3, we saw the activities of how midwives supported alternative physiological birth choices, however, the challenges highlighted for some study participants were mostly hidden. Indeed, women themselves may not be aware of any obstacles midwives face to support their decisions. Of course, women experiencing direct opposition, are acutely aware of the obstacles (Feeley & Thomson, 2016a), but where a midwife caregiver has willingly taken on their care, the women may be somewhat protected from tension and conflicts. Similarly for birth worker advocates or advocacy groups, while they express frustration at the lack of choices or barriers to getting women's needs met, they may not be aware of the emotional and mental labour (or the toll it takes) for midwives juxtaposed between the institution and woman (Big Birthas, 2021).[3] The obstacles or barriers can be overt (see later themes) or subtle as demonstrated in this emotion-story of 'feeling torn'. Torn between institutional working (shifts patterns, routines, expectations, political cultures) and women in their care, these accounts provide insights specifically around out of guidelines issues and broader issues of institutional routine care. Despite best efforts, the midwives' autonomy to deliver care aligned with their philosophy was limited and at times curtailed; creating some level of moral distress, related to the institutional, intra or inter-professional constraints placed upon them (Epstein & Hamric, 2009; King's Fund, 2020).

Limited agency and disrupted relationships were key factors in Katie's account when caring for a woman with a raised BMI wanting a homebirth. Significant tensions arose between Katie and her manager who felt the woman's decision-making was unsafe. Katie felt pressured to 'talk the woman' out of her decision and was deemed insubordinate for not doing so. Katie was in a marginalised position within the hierarchy, as a new member of staff to the team, and a junior, she felt judged to be incompetent rather than a midwife adhering to values of ethical competence (see Chapter 3). Torn between her manager, and her values to support the woman, this was a situation Katie could not win for the woman. The clashing of values led to a breakdown in trust, and following coercive strategies deployed by the manager, the woman opted out of maternity care altogether. Mirroring the wider research where some women or birthing people feel backed into a corner, they may disengage to freebirth (Feeley & Thomson, 2016b). Katie explains:

> … so I went to my manager who was already up in arms that this woman was going to have this homebirth with a BMI of 40 and also that she wouldn't speak to anybody else apart from me uhm, my manager was really unsupportive because she made out, because I was a junior member of the team, I hadn't managed to change this woman's mind, you know that I wasn't doing my job correctly, that I wasn't counselling her enough, you know I wasn't telling her about the risks enough, which I don't think was the case I think you know at the end of the day the woman had reached the end of her pregnancy, she knew what the risks were, you can't really bully anyone into doing, you can't frighten someone with all these things uhm my manager insisted I took another member of the community team to one of our appointments, which I did, but that really was the nail in the coffin for the woman's relationship with community midwives, and uhm she then after that she text me saying that she didn't trust me, that she wanted to freebirth and it was really stressful because all I wanted to do is support her, that really upset me because she obviously felt really cornered by everyone …

For Meg, her feelings of being torn permeated her interview through several examples. All had the same thread where Meg voiced deep concerns, moral compromise and distress (Litz & Kerig, 2019) as she felt strongly her organisational guidelines were not based on good evidence and were detrimental to women's experiences of care. Torn between her personal knowledge, competence and ethics and her employer's expectations to stay within guidelines, Meg expressed deep moral conflict. Bound by 'rules' and hierarchy, Meg struggled to consistently provide woman-centred care within its truest sense. Drawing upon one experience caring for someone during labour when it was discovered the baby was breech, Meg relayed her feelings of moral compromise as she stood beside the woman in theatre during the emergency caesarean, which Meg felt was unnecessary:

> … but basically uhm being in a theatre with this woman holding her hand as things were happening, and I just thought 'this shouldn't be happening' and I feel that as a I feel that as a terrible moral dilemma, it feels deeply immoral of me to uhm in a way, yes I feel it's a real dilemma …

Here Meg showed signs of moral distress (Jameton, 1984) due to her disagreement with the decision to perform an emergency caesarean (just) for a baby being breech. Rather than a tone of injustice, Meg's account was told with sadness and expressed internal conflict associated with feelings of complicity with the expectations of her employer, even though she did not share them. A cumulative effect as per Epstein & Hamric (2009) is evident as is a sense of moral injury. Her sense of immorality, a lack of agency and her loss of voice in speaking up, revealed self-blame and internalised failure (guilt and shame) rather than anger or resentment towards the structurally imposed limitations of institutional working (Litz & Kerig, 2019). Her struggle was also revealed below with long pauses between words, words trailing off and unfinished sentences[4]:

> … but also it does sound (..) my uhh (.) my responsibility as uhm (.) and my (..) uhh (.) my personal opinion as well especially what I feel to be right is conflicted to what my employer is expecting of me, that contractual, yea (..) that I find (..) really (…) that's difficult to live with that's (..) I feel I've (..) yea (..) I sometimes I have acted immoral, I feel powerless but (.) because I don't feel agency (..) within the situation (..) and then (.) then, and then in that dialogue with myself 'that's ridiculous' you know I am an experienced quite old person (laughs) I have a voice in my head (laughs) but my family were astonished that I wasn't quite able to speak up and those feelings were not (..) yea (..) of being difficult to speak (…) quite strong (..) and it's interesting that my family find that difficult to recognise (..)

Issues of incongruence between the guidelines, evidence and professional knowledge, were also found in Catherine's account. In her role as a senior midwife, she frequently counselled women about alternative physiological births. Recognising the tensions between the lack of evidence, (in this case, VBAC without continuous electronic fetal monitoring, yet numerous guidelines[5] are in favour of CEFM), and her own ethical competence, Catherine used subtle resistance to find a way to circumvent the tensions. Through careful use of language, Catherine met her employee obligations in discussing the local guidelines but created a way to instil messages of autonomy to subtly subvert the notion of guidelines as 'rules'. With the subtle language change seen below, Catherine becomes one step removed from the guidelines to align with the woman, creating the space for women to be the decision-maker. This is contextualised by her broader working environment where women's out of guideline care plans were reluctantly accepted (Feeley et al., 2019). Therefore, by 'toeing the line' and ensuring the local guidelines were discussed, she met the needs of the wider team and organisation, while maintaining support for women. As such she was able to navigate issues of moral compromise, avoiding deeply held moral distress as evident in other accounts:

> … I suppose I often say 'our guidelines suggest ' as opposed to 'I believe this' … this is what our guidelines suggest, it is a suggestion and not a 'this is protocol and we have to do it' sense to it, allowance, I hate that word, but it allows them to say 'I don't want to do that' …

A different perspective on feeling torn related to Margot's account, where she specifically stated she had a *'love-hate'* relationship with midwifery. She revealed she had feelings of love towards pregnant women and birth, emphasising the privilege she still felt and how she still cried at the birth of a baby, even after 17 years. Yet she equally hated the working conditions and environment she was in. Largely echoing broader issues of overwork, busyness, the administrative burden (King's Fund, 2020) and the broader political picture of austerity in the UK that has resulted in a fixed-term pay cut in the preceding ten years. However, during the interview, her brief mention of *'bitchiness'* revealed the bigger emotion-story. Intra-professional relationships had broken down, and personal conflicts had directly affected her in the workplace. Having *'been put in her place'* (by colleagues), Margot's account was one of isolation, having been ostracised by her colleagues, thus without a sense of belonging within her workplace (Geraghty et al., 2018; King's Fund, 2020):

> … I know my place and I will manage so I am very polite and friendly but I strongly feel that nobody there has got my back and that's a very lonely place a very lonely place …

When I asked Margot how she coped, she offered an uplifting account of leaning on her supportive and loving husband and family, as well as looking to the future with new life plans. However, this was also coupled with a sense of defensiveness:

> ... I'm not there to make friends, I'm not there to be popular, I'm there to do a job and earn my money and pay off my debts ...

Stories of battle

Building upon the stories of feeling torn, for other midwives, workplace stressors escalated with the metaphor of 'battle'. Barriers and obstacles are overt, vivid and frequent and while moral distress could occur and did take their mental/emotional toll, here, the midwives put up a fight. Compelled by a sense of duty towards women (and women's autonomy), their personal alignment towards physiological birth and evidence-based care, these passionate accounts of vocation and the pursuit of justice may have been a protective factor to succumbing to the effect of moral distress. The midwives positioned themselves as being in allegiance with the women, but against the 'system' that was perceived as unconducive to delivering woman-centred and/or evidence-based care. In these stories, we see advocacy and the deployment of knowledge practices. Knowledge was a 'weapon' to combat perceived inadequate care provision and to maintain ethically competent practice (see Chapter 3). Being knowledgeable was situated as both a source of frustration when knowledge clashed with their local culture/guidelines, and as a source of liberation when they used their wider knowledge to 'win' the battles. While the midwives maintained their ethical boundaries it does raise serious concerns around the sustainability of such an approach. With the potential impact of moral residue and the crescendo effect (Epstein & Hamric, 2009) without changes in their working environment, a profound long-term deleterious impact is likely.

Some experienced a *'daily battle'* with personal costs to their emotional and mental wellbeing alongside negative impacts on their family life. Some felt they had to *'pick their battles'* to maintain collegial relationships with their colleagues. Moreover, some felt stigmatised as a *'troublemaker'*, which manifested itself in two ways. One of these entailed feeling 'othered': *'not being part of the gang'*; resulting in social isolation and a reduced sense of belonging (King's Fund, 2020). A second manifestation related to fears they were perceived to be *'seen to be encouraging'* women's decision-making. To be perceived as influencing women's decisions appeared to put the midwives in a professionally vulnerable position. However, others positioned themselves with a *'reputation as a boat rocker'* reported with pride but also indicative of ongoing battles. The battles ranged from; intra-professional disputes such as conflicts and social isolation from midwifery colleagues to inter-professional disputes such as disagreements (even arguments) with medical colleagues, to broader institutional disputes where the guidelines appeared to impose authority over the midwives' practice and women's decision-making; or a combination of all three.

Jess' account was one of frustration. Infuriated by the injustice women's choices were frequently not respected (unless Jess advocated for them) and frustrated at a *'conveyor belt system'* of care. Here, Jess lamented the lack of individualised care despite the wider rhetoric to the contrary. Moreover, Jess challenged the idea women seeking out of guideline care were making 'riskier' choices. Reconstructing safety (as seen in Chapter 3), Jess relayed the statistics of her continuity team's service – cited as better than local and national averages, including the women who sought out of guidelines care. Jess's narrative constructions and countering of risk discourses are related to broader notions of 'good' and 'bad' mothering (Goodwin & Huppatz, 2010) and how this sociocultural construction plays out during women's birthing choices (Newnham, 2014). Her sense of injustice and frustration motivated her to fight for women:

> I felt so frustrated that this woman I cared for felt let down by the maternity services she initially engaged with. That she felt she was not being respected or listened to. She was just on a conveyor belt. A one size fits all approach doesn't work. It was sad that without having me as her advocate, she wouldn't have known that she could have made a plan with the SoM [Supervisor of Midwife][6] and consultant midwife. She probably wouldn't have had a positive, natural birth. I feel frustrated that it feels like a constant daily battle to support women who choose to go 'off guideline'. It is expected that women will do what they are told as the guidelines and health professionals know best. I know that we have to constantly risk assess every decision and that we want a healthy mum and a healthy baby, and that safety is paramount. But, we forget that it's that pregnant woman and her partner's decision to make, not ours. Women don't tend to choose to put themselves or their babies at risk. But risk is relative and individual.

Moreover, Jess' battles appeared to have culminated in a feeling of 'us and them' (Link & Phelan, 2001) due to being labelled as a *'troublemaker'* by her labour ward[7] midwifery colleagues who perceived Jess as 'brainwashing' women into making out of guidelines birth choices. Such a clash of ethical perspectives, where Jess may be perceived as acting unethically, is a professionally dangerous position to be in. Here, the disparity between the rhetoric of woman-centred care and informed choices and the reality of practice is stark:

> I often feel like I am labelled as a 'troublemaker' midwife when I walk on labour ward. That people think I am brainwashing my women to decline induction or decline prophylactic antibiotics etc. when in reality I am just supporting them to make their own informed decisions. Once women realise that they have choice and a voice, they feel more confident to do what feels right for them in their own unique circumstances.

While Jess is maintaining her ethical boundaries to manage the potential moral compromise, the long-term sustainability of her approach is in question. Frequent conflicts within the workplace are a known stressor which can lead to burnout (Geraghty et al., 2018; Hunter et al., 2019). Similarly, Alex (in Chapter 3) also met the challenge of maintaining ethical boundaries to resist moral compromise. Where Alex was supporting a woman with Group B Strep within her local birth centre she navigated power struggles between several layers of the maternity system whereby conflicting population-level evidence was used as a method of persuasion for individual women (see Chapter 2). In the case she described, the woman's decision appeared to be systemically marginalised. Although Alex did 'eventually' manage to negotiate the woman's entry to the birth centre as previously discussed (page 60), this birth choice was only enabled because Alex agreed to be personally on call for the woman, as it was felt unfair on other midwives to take the (perceived) risk of caring for the woman concerned. Since this entailed being on call for some weeks there is a concern about work-life balance and sustainability for individual midwives who try to support women's choices against such systemic opposition (Crowther et al., 2016). Without institutional support for the woman's birth plan, and the onus is on a particular midwife, an undue emotional burden and responsibility is placed upon an individual, whereas a shared collective responsibility to meet the needs of birthing women and people is essential for psychological safety and wellbeing (King's Fund, 2020). Furthermore, had Alex not been able to go on call this could have been a morally compromising situation (Litz & Kerig, 2019).

Power struggles were also evident in Seana's account where she disagreed with an obstetric doctor's insistence to intervene with syntocinon[8] for what Seana felt was a woman progressing normally in labour. Seana's broader narrative of ongoing battles related to the tension between a particularly medicalised workplace where she was perceived as a 'radical' midwife going against local norms. Situated as a 'lone ranger', Seana worked to engineer changes toward physiological evidence-based birth practices. Whilst still an ongoing battle, Seana reported some change was occurring:

> … its having an impact. Rather than me being a lone ranger, which I was for a long time, I can see subtle change, even simple things like delayed cord clamping. Some midwives were like 'why would you bother?' and I'm like 'oh my god' so I would go and print out an article and leave it on the kitchen table or whatever. And now to hear people talking, rather than me being the mouthpiece all the time …

In contrast to Alex's account, it appeared Seana had some level of support– although this was variable depending on whether her colleagues 'got her'. Those who understood Seana appeared to 'let her get on with it' thus suggesting to have autonomy, she needed to be understood and respected. Similarly, Stella reported being supported by her direct managers but did report confrontations and conflicts with other colleagues. In particular, she described *'loathing'* transfers from homebirths to the obstetric unit due to poor working relationships between her team and the hospital colleagues. Being labelled as one with a 'reputation' for speaking out, was felt to be the source of tension. These could be seen as situations of moral conflict and while the midwives in this section appear to have maintained their ethical values, we must ask, at what cost?

The toll of continued battles was particularly evident in Edna's broader narrative -overburdened by the responsibility for women's outcomes and more so the women's experience, especially if women did not get their choices facilitated by other maternity professionals. More so, Edna's stress related to the professional vulnerability supporting alternative choices exposed her to. Confident within her ethical competence, it was not intrapartum caregiving that was problematic, rather the fears of 'finger pointing' within a blame culture (Robertson & Thomson, 2016) created such a toll:

> … uhm if I'm honest I don't think it's the fear that anything is going to go wrong brutally because actually I am not going to put a woman in that position, I am not going to put myself in that position, it's the fear of finger pointing, it's the fear of being hauled up in front of the Trust organisation and saying and them saying that you didn't do all that you could, you didn't talk her out of it, I hate that, you get that a lot, 'why can't you talk her out of it.

The combination of the emotional burden of women's outcomes and fear of reprisals placed a significant mental and emotional toll on Edna. When I asked how she managed, she shared the impact upon her emotional and mental wellbeing, running counter to the King's Fund (2020) recommendations:

> … but I don't think I do manage it if I'm honest, my mental health suffers because of it, my family life suffers because of it uhm and everyone is the same, I'm not in isolation from that point of view, but I do, I lose sleep at night because of these women, I do, we all suffer with anxiety, I'd say 50% of the midwives that practice in the same way as I do suffer because of the effort and the strain it puts on everything …

However, for two midwives, while they did experience battles, they did have some 'protection' from the negative impacts of recurring conflicts. These two midwives worked in 'like-minded' teams wherein ongoing mutual support provided a source of resilience. Strong, positive and close-knit teams helped manage the potential moral compromising situations and conflicts, thus, largely avoiding moral distress. While there was a sense of 'us and them' where the midwives (and their immediate teams) were in frequent conflict with the wider hospital team; the midwives did have their core needs met through their immediate teams. Autonomy, working within their values, belonging and a sense of contribution

(King's Fund, 2020) were cultivated via their immediate teams, sustaining them to maintain the provision of woman-centred care:

> … when you go and you've had a birth on labour ward and I come home questioning myself 'was I too bolshy? did I come across like this? could I have phrased that a bit better?' when I'm anxious to speak up I probably come across quite angry because I am a little bit, talking a bit fast am a bit flushed, and you go back to your team and they go 'no come on that sounds like you did the right thing, you had to say something, well done you for speaking up, it takes a lot to speak up' so you think ok I did the right thing which is exactly what you need because I think you probably wouldn't let go of those feelings, and also we get to see the women afterwards that makes a difference for us as well, we get to speak to them and get their feedback and maybe they say 'thank you for speaking up about that' or whatever, or maybe they don't (laughs).

Stories of reproach, recrimination or vilification

Building on the stories of battle, the narratives of three participants could be viewed as examples of the battle almost lost. All three participants experienced a formal investigation of their midwifery practice. In two situations, this was due to poor fetal outcomes whereby later, the midwives were exonerated. The other case investigated was due to concerns that CEFM was not used (but where there was no adverse fetal outcome). In all three situations, the midwives reported supporting and facilitating the woman's decision-making, guided by their midwifery philosophy of woman-centred care and wider professional knowledge. Although the poor outcomes were distressing, they were not issues of morality or negligence. Rather, the moral injury occurred by the reaction from their employing organisations, deploying a punitive approach to investigating the incidents. While adverse outcomes do need to be investigated, the nature and conduct of investigations are variable across the NHS (Robertson & Thomson, 2016). For these midwives, they felt the investigations and/or referral to the Nursing and Midwifery Council[9] were unduly punitive, and an opportunity to scapegoat the individual midwives. Mirroring Smith's (2021) findings of moral injury caused by *'cruel neglect and rejection'* (p. 37) from peers following a serious incident, these accounts were constructed through stories of isolation and marginalisation contextualised by a blame culture within their working environments.

For Leanne,[10] while she was vindicated of any wrongdoing, the investigation process left a significant mark on her mental and emotional wellbeing, detrimentally affecting her midwifery practice, and created disillusionment in the notion of woman-centred care. So much so, Leanne was making plans to leave the profession at the time of the interview. During the immense level of scrutiny that is associated with punitive investigations (Robertson & Thomson, 2016), Leanne lost all confidence in her clinical skills and lacked support to overcome the psychological distress of being involved in a tragic case where neonatal death occurred. Moreover, the investigation completely undermined her confidence in midwifery (and the rhetorical philosophy of woman-centred care) in the broader sense. She was reprimanded for not coercing the woman to accept a vaginal examination. This was in direct opposition to her midwifery philosophy, in which she viewed advocacy and respecting informed consent as an inherent role of the midwife, and to deny such, is abuse:

> … My colleagues and supervisor of midwives have advised me that I should be 'more forceful', or get another midwife into the room to 'help convince the woman'. However, I strongly believe that consent is a choice and, if you have thoroughly explained what you want to do and the rationale behind why you want to do it, if the woman does not want you to do whatever it is, you do not do it otherwise it is not consent and could be classed as abuse.

The conflict between her sense of midwifery, morality and her experiences of the investigation exposed a wider incongruence in the rhetoric of a midwives' role and the reality of what happens (in some places) when things go wrong. In this situation, moral distress and injury were related to institutional blame punitively questioning her decision-making during the episode of care (Smith, 2021). This runs counter to an open, learning culture where maternity professionals are supported psychologically and clinically throughout adverse events and subsequent investigations (Smith, 2021). Remembering Leanne was vindicated of wrongdoing, the reaction by senior midwives insisting Leanne should have been more 'forceful' with the woman highlighted the incongruence between the values of woman-centred care and reality. For Leanne, there was a strong sense of loss, of midwifery not being what she had been taught it to be:

> Yes, it just completely undermined, it showed that midwifery is more about protecting your back than it is advocating for women. And that in itself is just very very sad because as a student going into midwifery, you expect it to be(e) (emphasis) to be all about women and advocating for women and fighting their corner. But actually, when it comes to the grindstone, when it comes to the crunch, it is not about advocating for women, it is about protecting your back …

Moreover, Leanne constructed the investigation as one of a personal attack on her midwifery practice. The inference was had she been aligned with intuitional norms rather than the woman, then she would have escaped blame:

> … when things go wrong, it is the midwife who they look to destroy. It does not seem to matter if you were advocating for that family or supporting their choices at the time, even though all things seemed normal then. It seems to matter if you covered your back with vigilant documentation, if

the woman 'did as she was told', and how well you, as a midwife, can stand up and fight for yourself and your practice.

A strong sense of disillusionment was also apparent for Beatrice.[11] However, for Beatrice, rather than sadness, she was *'burning with rage'* – influenced by her perceptions that institutionalised maternity practices have increasingly *'infantilised the role of the midwife and that of pregnant women'.* Such infantilisation appeared to play out in her experience of supervised practice[12] where she felt a disparity between a midwives' autonomous practice and the evidence base, the institutionalised routine use of guidelines, toxic organisational norms, and a subservient culture. Beatrice was clear in her reasons for joining the study, and voiced strong political concerns about the nature of midwifery and maternity services:

> I chose to share this story as an antidote to anger and resentment. I became a midwife because I wanted to protect and enhance women's health and their rights. It feels more and more that I am ensnared in a mad conspiracy which licenses obstetric butchery. Failure to comply with the legislation or the requisite guidelines results in professional vilification. The joke of the matter is that in terms of evidence-based practice, CEFM [continuous electronic fetal monitoring] has little to recommend it and certainly not for a healthy primip with a normal Body Mass Index and blood glucose levels.

Beatrice's anger and frustration, represented by sarcasm, exposed power and authority struggles between both herself as a midwife and obstetrics but also the marginalisation of women making their own decisions. With similarities with 'good' and 'bad' mother sociocultural constructions (Goodwin & Huppatz, 2010), Beatrice's' narrative suggested a notion of the 'good' and 'bad' midwife- where the 'bad' midwife is responsible for women making *'bad'* choices:

> Like Don Quixote de la Mancha, I tilt at the windmills that declare women are weak, midwives are subservient to obstetricians and need to be stripped of the vestiges of professional autonomy ... Perhaps I have fallen down a rabbit hole where every pregnant woman is too stupid and weak to make her own choices, form her own birth plan and see it through. Perhaps it is right that a consultant obstetrician should hector an experienced midwife who is – after all – responsible for a woman making a 'bad' choice.

Behind Beatrice's anger and indignation, was also a deeply distressing account of her experiences in supervised practice. During the interview, I tentatively asked whether she would like to talk about the experience, and within her responses, she revealed a devastating account of its impact – a moral injury occurred. Central to this was being removed from the clinical area in which the complaint arose, and the subsequent social isolation this caused. Such a punitive approach caused a strong sense of *'shame'* that she has not *'got over'* indicating the extent of her psychological distress. As such, Beatrice constructed her experience as a *'watershed moment'* which had far-reaching consequences across her whole life; her sense of identity, loss of friends and work colleagues, damage to her career, poor mental and emotional wellbeing, and a detrimental financial impact.[13] However, fortunately for Beatrice, she reported finding solace in family and friends. Additionally, through the kindness of other colleagues, she was helped through the process of completing her required hours, enabling her to stay in the profession.

In a similar experience, Georgina had several examples of confrontations with midwifery and obstetric colleagues disagreeing with her midwifery practice of supporting women's decisions. Georgina reported feeling *'attacked with ferocity'* during an altercation where it was suggested she was *'brainwashing women'*. Georgina reported several challenging situations where she received little support from midwifery and obstetric colleagues, giving rise to a toxic working environment. She reported being *'scapegoated'* for a poor outcome during a breech birth. Several intra-professional conflicts occurred whilst the local investigation was carried out and was felt to catalyse a referral to the NMC. Whilst the outcome was *'no case to answer'*,[14] it was a *'threatening and traumatic'* time. Like Beatrice, Georgina found support in midwifery colleagues, but only in those external to her hospital. This support was crucial to Georgina remaining a midwife. Despite numerous conflicts, Georgina's broader self-reflective narrative revealed her beliefs that her midwifery practice had a higher purpose. As a midwife with international expertise and a unique skill set, Georgina referred to how she could *'weather the storms'*. Through a mixture of acceptance that poor outcomes will occur, and recognition that she is likely to be targeted in future, Georgina also believed these storms reflected what is wrong with the system. Constructing social deviance as a positive gave her the strength to continue as a midwife:

> … like I said that is part of the work I do I just get back up again, and someone somewhere will attempt to knock me down, to a certain extent sometimes I don't even take it personal, you know I just think it's, it is just a manifestation of all that is wrong with the system and me taking the moral high ground and just carrying on just doing what I do is part of challenging that system.

Unmet needs, wounded midwives

This chapter has shown the negative impact on midwives endeavouring to deliver woman-centred care within working environments with opposing values. The negative experiences are characterised by a misalignment between the midwives' ethical values and philosophy and their employing organisation. Collectively, the midwives' experiences showed degrees of moral compromise, distress and for a few, moral injury (Litz & Kerig, 2019). Viewed within the King's Fund framework (2020), we can see the midwives primarily experienced challenges to autonomous working and acting *consistently* within their values. For some midwives, issues of belonging were apparent – disconnection with colleagues, and feeling unvalued or supported had a significant impact on their emotional and mental wellbeing. Navigating issues of contribution, all had a strong need to be effective in their work, delivering woman-centred alternative physiological birth care and practicing 'full-scope midwifery'. Largely, they did achieve this, and for many, it was their alignment and allegiance with women which fostered a strong sense of contribution. However, for some midwives in these accounts, it came at a great cost. High levels of emotional labour and mental load created undue stress and/or distress and are akin to psychologically unsafe work environments. This is significant in terms of sustainability, for ongoing and sustained distress has far-reaching mental, emotional and physical implications impacting workforce sustainability. In the next chapter, the opposite is presented – midwives working in supportive, psychologically safe environments, so much so that they were flourishing in their job.

Notes

1 Much of these concepts were developed by researchers focusing on war veterans but since then it has become a growing field across a number of domains including healthcare – see special issue (Litz & Kerig, 2019). In midwifery, it is a growing area of interest (Foster et al., 2022). However, it is important to recognise that the empirical field related to these concepts is undergoing rapid growth and development as researchers from a range of disciplines have turned their attention to this area (Litz & Kerig, 2019). In terms of clinical applications some definitions may change, be amended, however for the purposes of a qualitative inquiry such as this book, the conceptualisations offer useful tools to understand the midwives negative and distressing experiences of delivering alternative physiological birth care.

2 Different authors use moral distress and injury interchangeably however, I concur with Litz and Kerig (2010) that the continuum model with the three core terms compromise, distress and injuy as the most useful heuristically to covey the nuance of experience and subsequent psychological impact.

3 On reflection, now approaching publication of this book, I feel this statement is less true as there is greater awareness around midwives' morally compromised situations thanks to campaigns such as March with Midwives.

4 For the purposes of this extract, I have kept the pauses in the text, denoted by (.) for one second pause (..) for two etc. I felt it was important to convey the difficulty Meg had in expressing herself, primarily because she was deeply saddened by the situation.

5 Continuous electronic fetal monitoring (CEFM) for women wanting a vaginal birth after caesarean is an ongoing contentious issue. All major organisations in the UK including RCOG and NICE recommend its use, where NICE acknowledges there is no sound evidence in favour of CEFM during VBAC (NICE, 2019). During NICE's most recent consultation they had removed this recommendation but following the consultation it was reinstated.

6 In the UK, we no longer have Supervisor of Midwives as this was removed from statute, see Chapter 1 for insights.

7 Labour ward is also known as the obstetric unit or delivery suite.

8 Artificial hormone drip used to speed up labour.

9 Investigations are often carried out by the in-house organisational teams, but where concerns are raised about a midwife's fitness to practice, they can be referred to the NMC for further investigation, with the potential to be struck off the register.

10 For Leanne, she was providing intrapartum care to a woman with an uncomplicated pregnancy and labour. When offered a vaginal examination to assess cervical

progress, the woman not so much declined outright but asked for it to be done later. In Leanne's assessment all other observations remained within normal parameters until the head was visible, a prolonged deceleration prompted a transfer to the obstetric unit where the baby was born in poor condition. The baby later died. Such an unexpected adverse outcome clearly warrants an investigation, however, the nature of the investigation as Leanne described in her interview was poorly handled and created extreme psychological distress. Furthermore, the investigation exonerated her practice, she had acted in accordance to the clinical picture at the time and escalated appropriately at the first sign of fetal compromise.

11 Beatrice was caring for a woman with diet-controlled gestational diabetes who had gone into spontaneous labour, requesting the pool. Beatrice's hospital guidelines recommended continuous electronic fetal monitoring which was not available with the pool. Beatrice reported counselling the woman on benefits and risks, including inquiring whether the woman would be prepared to leave the pool if intermittent auscultation highlighted any concerns (to which consent was sought and gained). There were no clinical concerns throughout the labour, Beatrice provided 1:1 care throughout and no later adverse outcome. However, the woman not having CEFM was met with poor reactions from the wider team, to which, a complaint was put in against Beatrice.

12 When a midwife has been referred to the NMC they can put restrictions on their practice, including having 'supervised practice' akin to being a student where your practice is continually monitored and assessed by other midwives. If the midwife fails to meet the core competencies it would result in being struck off. Otherwise, at the end of supervised practice, the midwife can then remain on the professional register.

13 Whilst on supervised practice, Beatrice could not work extra shifts or work for agencies.

14 An NMC finding which meant no further actions are required, no supervision required, and the midwife can remain on the register.

References

Big Birthas. (2021). *Midwives Supporting Alternative Birth Choices – New Research!* https://www.bigbirthas.co.uk/midwives-supporting-alternative-birth-choices/

Crowther, S., Hunter, B., McAra-Couper, J., Warren, L., Gilkison, A., Hunter, M., Fielder, A., & Kirkham, M. (2016). Sustainability and resilience in midwifery: A discussion paper. *Midwifery*, 40, 40–48. doi: 10.1016/j.midw.2016.06.005

Epstein, E., & Hamric, A. (2009). Moral distress, moral residue, and the crescendo effect. *The Journal of Clinical Ethics*, 20(4), 330–342.

Feeley, C., & Thomson, G. (2016a). Tensions and conflicts in 'choice': Women's' experiences of freebirthing in the UK. *Midwifery*, 41, 16–21. doi: 10.1016/j.midw.2016.07.014

Feeley, C., & Thomson, G. (2016b). Why do some women choose to freebirth in the UK? An interpretative phenomenological study. *BMC Pregnancy and Childbirth*, 16, 59. doi: 10.1186/s12884-016-0847-6

Feeley, C., Thomson, G., & Downe, S. (2019). Caring for women making unconventional birth choices: A meta-ethnography exploring the views, attitudes, and experiences of midwives. *Midwifery*, 72, 50–59. doi: 10.1016/j.midw.2019.02.009

Foster, W., McKellar, L., Fleet, J., & Sweet, L. (2022). Moral distress in midwifery practice: A concept analysis. *Nursing Ethics*, 29(2), 364–383. doi: 10.1177/09697330211023983

Fourie, C. (2017). Who is experiencing what kind of moral distress? Distinctions for moving from a narrow to a broad definition of moral distress. *AMA Journal of Ethics*, 19(6), 578–584. doi: 10.1001/journalofethics.2017.19.6.nlit1–1706

Geraghty, S., Speelman, C., & Bayes, S. (2018). Fighting a losing battle: Midwives experiences of workplace stress. *Women Birth*, 32(3), e297–e306. doi: 10.1016/j.wombi.2018.07.012

Goodwin, S., & Huppatz, K. E. (2010). The good mother in theory and research: An overview. In S. Goodwin, & K. Huppatz (Eds.), *The Good Mother: Contemporary Motherhoods in Australia* (pp. 1–24). Sydney University Press.

Hunter, B., Fenwick, J., Sidebotham, M., & Henley, J. (2019). Midwives in the United Kingdom: Levels of burnout, depression, anxiety and stress and associated predictors. doi: 7910.1016/j.midw.2019.08.008

Jameton, A. (1984). *Nursing Practice: The Ethical Issues*. Prentice Hall.

King's Fund. (2020). *The Courage of Compassion: Supporting Nurses and Midwives to Deliver High-Quality Care*. London: King's Fund. https://www.kingsfund.org.uk/sites/default/files/2020-09/The%20courage%20of%20compassion%20full%20report_0.pdf

Kleres, J. (2011). Emotions and narrative analysis: A methodological approach. *Journal for the Theory of Social Behaviour*, 41(2), 182–202. doi: 10.1111/j.1468–5914.2010.00451.x

Link, B. G., & Phelan, J. C. (2001). Conceptualizing stigma. *Annual Review of Sociology*, 27(1), 363–385. doi: 10.1146/annurev.soc.27.1.363

Litz, B., & Kerig, P. (2019). Introduction to the special issue on moral injury: Conceptual challenges, methodological issues, and clinical applications. *Journal of Traumatic Stress*, 32(3), 341–349. doi: 10.1002/jts.22405

Newnham, E. (2014). Birth control: Power/knowledge in the politics of birth. *Health Sociology Review*, 23(3), 254–268. doi: 10.1080/14461242.2014.11081978

NICE. (2019). *Intrapartum Care for Women with Existing Medical Conditions or Obstetric Complications and Their Babies*. London: NICE. https://www.nice.org.uk/guidance/ng121/chapter/recommendations

Robertson, J. H., & Thomson, A. M. (2016). An exploration of the effects of clinical negligence litigation on the practice of midwives in England: A phenomenological study. *Midwifery*, 33, 55–63. doi: 10.1016/j.midw.2015.10.005

Smith, J. (2021). *Nurturing maternity staff: How to tackle trauma, stress and burnout to create a positive working culture in the NHS*. Pinter & Martin: London.

5

PSYCHOLOGICALLY SAFE WORK ENVIRONMENTS

Creating the conditions for fulfilment

The previous chapter introduced the second analysis conducted in this study; using the lens of 'emotionality', rich insights into the midwives' experiences of supporting alternative physiological birth were captured. Chapter 4 highlighted the varying degrees of challenges for some of the midwives, conceptualised by moral compromise, distress and injury. Arguably, those midwives worked in psychologically *unsafe* environments. In this chapter, psychologically safe environments are examined, through which, other emotion-stories are revealed. Two different aspects were found; first, the change-maker midwives demonstrated compassionate leadership to facilitate the evolution of institutional culture towards greater woman-centredness, enhancing psychologically safe workplaces – 'Stories of transition'. Second, in direct comparison to the previous chapter, 'Stories of fulfilment' captures the emotions, feelings and experiences of midwives working within psychologically safe environments. Broadly these environments cultivated feelings of normalcy when supporting alternative physiological births – the midwives could 'just get on with the job'. Moreover, these enabling environments created the space for some to experience awe, wonder and the sublime. Collectively, these storylines provide hope and optimism – with the right support structures in place, supporting and facilitating these births can be a joy and a source of fulfilment.

Emotion stories: Psychologically safe, enabling environments

Chapter 4 demonstrated constraints within the midwives' ability to support alternative physiological birthing choices. Furthermore, as per the King's Fund (2020) ABC model differing aspects of autonomy, belonging and contribution were affected by misalignments between the midwives and their workplace

DOI: 10.4324/9781003265443-5

environments. Conversely, when these needs are met, staff engagement (with organisational goals and person-centred care), greater wellbeing and flourishing are enhanced (King's Fund, 2020). Crucially, staff wellbeing is strongly correlated with safety outcomes, and is vital for safe, high-quality care (West et al., 2014; West et al., 2017). Where top-down and system-wide organisational cultures are characterised by mutual respect, support and trust, job satisfaction and enjoyment occur (King's Fund, 2020). Such cultures can be viewed as 'enabling environments' (RCPSYCH, 2020); where midwives are trusted to work autonomously and to the fullest extent of midwifery practice, they are less likely to leave the profession (Hunter et al., 2018; RCM, 2016). Moreover, a positive workplace culture influences midwives' sense of 'social capital' – the strength of connection between themselves and colleagues (Hunter, 2010). Horizontal trust (employee to employee) and reciprocity facilitate these connections (Hunter, 2010). Other maternity research has highlighted positive collegial relationships, and in some cases, akin to being a family – promoting flexible working, mutual support and friendships as essential ingredients to support midwifery workforce sustainability (Hunter, 2010; Walsh, 2007).[1] Critically, these positive working environments are characterised by high levels of psychological safety.

Psychological safety was first defined by Edmondson (1999) as 'a shared belief held by team members that the team is safe for interpersonal risk-taking' (p. 350). The relationships between team members give rise to tacit and explicit social expectations (culture) of what is and is not acceptable (Edmondson, 1999). In a psychologically safe culture, interrelationships are based on positive, trusting and respectful behaviour between team members (Edmondson, 1999; O'Donovan & McAuliffe, 2020). This includes the space to voice mistakes, differences of opinion or even disagreements – safe within the knowledge it will be received well (not punitively). Brown (2018) refers to the ability to have hard, uncomfortable conversations which are kind, clear and respectful with the space for shared vulnerabilities. These points are critical in healthcare teams who are working within a fast-paced, complex and high-stakes environment, and where those individuals need to work interdependently to coordinate safe care (Nembhard & Edmondson, 2006; O'Donovan & McAuliffe, 2020), particularly pertinent for those supporting alternative physiological births. However, for psychological safety to be operationalised it must be embedded within a learning, not blaming culture. Accepting mistakes will occur in such busy complex environments and supporting staff through those occasions are central to fostering openness and honesty and improving overall patient safety outcomes (Nembhard & Edmondson, 2006; O'Donovan & McAuliffe, 2020). Related to the analysis of team dynamics, Edmondson (1999) refers to 'learning behaviour' which as seen below, requires psychological safety to operationalise:

> the ongoing process of reflection and action, characterized by asking questions, seeking feedback, experimenting, reflecting on results, and discussing errors or unexpected outcomes of actions. (p. 353)

Such learning behaviour requires a system-wide learning culture embedded throughout an organisation; therefore, good leadership is required (Nembhard & Edmondson, 2006; West et al., 2017). Compassionate leadership behaviours such as attending, understanding, empathising and helping the staff, create psychologically safe environments (Edmondson, A. & Harvey, 2017). This approach differs from the 'command and control' approach that dominates some workplaces; known to silence staff voices, suppress new and creative ideas and suffocate intrinsic motivation (West & Bailey, 2019). Conversely, compassionate leadership encourages creativity, sharing of ideas and positive interrelationships, in turn, facilitates a shared vision and a collective focus on high-quality care (West & Bailey, 2019). Moreover, where staff are empowered to participate within a collective leadership model, led by compassionate leadership, it fosters a sense of belonging, ownership, and shared responsibility (West et al., 2014). Through visible, compassionate leadership, where proactive support is demonstrated by upper-level management, psychological safety is enhanced and reinforced through trusting relationships (West et al., 2014); thus, encouraging greater 'interpersonal risk-taking' where speaking up, raising concerns or having greater confidence to work outside of comfort zones are more likely (Edmondson, 1999). To be a compassionate leader requires high levels of courage, resilience, and beliefs along with commitment to enacting the principles (West & Bailey, 2019). These positive effects of compassionate, collective leadership are seen throughout this chapter. However, first, the midwives demonstrate the (hard) work involved to create psychologically safe workplaces demonstrating the important emotional labour required to improve birthing women and people's access to care of their choosing. In the second part of the chapter, the midwives highlight the positive experiences of working within established psychologically safe workplaces, whereby the midwives were supported to facilitate alternative physiological births.

Stories of transition

This overarching storyline traverses the '*Stories of distress*' and '*Stories of fulfilment*' where some of the midwives were the 'change makers' within their organisation. All within leadership positions, their goal and purpose was to improve the culture toward greater woman-centredness which included improved access to and the delivery of alternative physiological birth care. Accordingly, they were responsible for driving institutional change using different leadership approaches including compassionate and collective leadership to support the 'buy-in' from the staff. Such buy-in was essential as the participants overcame significant resistance to improving access to women's alternative choices. Resistance regarding concerns of safety and/or liability stemmed from both midwife caregivers, obstetrics and the organisations. However, often it was reported the midwife caregivers[2] were particularly fearful of '*widening the criteria*' of women who can be supported in low-risk settings. Such fears were recounted in relation to '*losing their PIN*' (registration), and/or being scapegoated in the event of a poor outcome

– echoing earlier storylines in Chapter 4. Therefore, the job of these participants was to provide proactive and meaningful support to garner trust (the buy-in) so the midwife caregivers believed they had the backing of the organisation during alternative physiological birthcare.

As such, the accounts revealed the extensive nature of such work to bring about the 'buy-in' required to foster systemic changes. To facilitate changes, the work involved comprehensive negotiations across all professional groups and often within challenging hierarchical structures. However, the participants were in leadership roles, contributing to levelling power imbalances within such structures. Developing and asserting professional '*clout*' appeared to be an asset to enhance perceptions of authority. Professional clout required '*proving*' themselves to women and all professional groups as knowledgeable and competent. Collectively, the nature of such work indicated an extensive mental load. Some participants felt this was '*unseen*' work which was difficult to '*measure*', and therefore, sometimes devalued. However, highlighting change was '*moving on*', Tracey revealed a tipping point was reached following extensive work carried out by a senior team with support from the Head of Midwifery (HoM). Tracey reported extensive negotiations and collaborations with the multidisciplinary team over a long period resulted in significant changes to the delivery suite guidelines and the criteria for women's choices were broadened. The widened criteria were perceived as '*unreal*' denoting a sense of surprisingly progressive change, in comparison to the previous restrictive guidelines:

> … so now they've changed, just recently they have just put out a draft guideline and the criteria for women on delivery suite who can go on now is unreal, I mean the midwives are now like 'oh what?' cos they've said that IUD[3] ladies can use the pool, and the midwives are like 'why would you let them?' and I'm like 'well why not?' … but they've [obstetricians/risk and governance teams] gone like the other way.

From a different perspective, Jenna's account provided a vivid insight into the speed at which systemic changes could occur. Jenna talked at great length about the positive changes occurring during the short 18 months she had been in a leadership position. Exploring how this occurred so quickly, she attributed a combination of dogged determination, the importance of creating a '*safe*' non-punitive environment for the midwife caregivers, alongside simultaneous wider cultural changes in the organisation. Thus, Jenna's organisation reached a cultural change tipping point relatively quickly. Central to which was creating trusting relationships with her colleagues and the midwife caregivers, enhancing the psychological safety within the organisation (Edmondson, 1999; West et al., 2017):

> It is quick, and it's about you, I can't say it enough, it's about you uhm people have to see you doing what you say you're going to do number one, number two they have to feel safe, I call it professional safety, people have

to feel safe in the role in they're doing, they have to know if they follow their role and what's expected of them, they can't be touched in a negative way, they need to know that otherwise they won't do what you're asking them to do because they're too frightened.

Moreover, Jenna drew upon her previous experience within the same organisation, recognising previous issues of a punitive working culture had been detrimental to women getting their needs met and the midwives feeling supported (Robertson & Thomson, 2016). She reflected and claimed her own sense of accountability, recognising her role in perpetuating a punitive working environment. These experiences appeared to have facilitated personal growth, coinciding with new conceptual understandings of human factors[4] and psychologically safe work environments:

> they've got to be safe, the woman has got to be safe but the midwife has got to be safe, the worst thing you can see if a midwife has a poor outcome … that's why we've moved on in this trust, there was a lot of punitive action I feel, it was the system, I was a part of that system, I was definitely a part of that system because I came in as a matron, this is what you do, everybody is doing it, this is what you're supposed to do then over the years I thought 'no, there is something not right here, something not quite right' and that's where the human factors came in, human factors and complex birth is beautiful together …

Jenna described the changes as an *'evolution'* where she anticipated (and had evidence of) midwife caregivers becoming more receptive to supporting women's alternative birthing decisions. A key element of her success appeared to be her willingness to collaborate with her teams. Through a collective, compassionate leadership approach, Jenna valued the community midwives as *'experts'* in their respective fields, and as such, the care plans were devised collaboratively. Meaningful collaboration appeared to have instilled more confidence in the midwife caregivers to write the care plans, and to take ownership and a shared responsibility (West et al., 2014), culminating in less *'reliance'* on Jenna. Jenna's example captures the essence of compassionate leadership and the positive impact of creating psychologically safe environments for the midwife caregivers; shifting the management culture and style was crucial to harnessing trust in the caregivers they were genuinely supported. Moreso, moving to a democratised, collective leadership approach, Jenna found the midwife caregivers increasingly prepared to take 'interpersonal risks' (Edmondson, 1999) and responsibility (West et al., 2014). Furthermore, seeking their views as experts in their own right in their clinical area fostered being valued with something to contribute (King's Fund, 2020):

> … so I will say to the community midwives 'this is the plan, do you think it will work, is it feasible? And if not, what do you think will work?' And

gradually, I get emails all the time now like 'this lady wants a homebirth and I think we can do a, b, c, d but I'm not sure about' and I'm thinking 'yes' before I would just get emails 'this woman wants a homebirth, can you go see her?' it's starting now to synthesise some of the stuff that I am feeding them so they're not so reliant I think …

Collectively, the midwives in this storyline facilitated change through compassionate leadership styles, working in extensive collaboration with the multi-disciplinary team and midwifery caregivers (as opposed to top-down directives). However, the change agents had to provide meaningful structures, tacit and practical, to overcome resistance from midwife caregivers. Visual artefacts such as care pathways or guidelines or care plans endorsed by the organisation combined with direct support from the change agents were key to fostering trusting relationships and psychologically safe environments:

Yea, so the supervisors used to do the care plan but they were uhm they, they probably weren't written as well as they could have been, they probably didn't include the discussion around the actual evidence … it's definitely bringing a consultant midwife in with her training uhm that formalised those care plans and made them a lot more professional and acceptable to the medical team uhm and the learning that and I also think it is something that is quite easily taught so uhm … We've run it past our legal department now as well to say how does this affect our insurance, does this look like a robust enough letter? And they're really really happy with it.

[Jenny]

Stories of fulfilment

Building on the '*Stories of transition*', the narratives in this storyline from 20 participants conveyed the other side of the process, where sufficient cultural shifts had occurred, and change was embedded. Where there were multiple levels of conflict and subsequent moral compromise or distress in Chapter 4, here we see something entirely different; the accounts were marked by a lack of conflict, animosity or distress, and the workplace is de-centred in their stories, giving rise to new emotion-stories. For some this was related to a sense of the 'ordinary', where a feeling of being able to 'get on' with the job of facilitating women's choices was identified. This was associated with the midwives being situated within supportive working environments where women's alternative choices were mostly accepted. For others, their narratives related to a sense of camaraderie either between themselves and the woman or themselves and their team. Finally, the other participants expressed a feeling of the sublime, through accounts of love, awe, tenderness, attunement and reverence.

Stories of normalised practice

The normalcy of supporting alternative physiological birth choices could be described for 10 midwives as simply as midwives enabled to get on with the job, practising 'full-scope' midwifery (Renfrew et al., 2014) and secure in the knowledge that they were supported by their employing organisation. While they may have experienced resistance from *some* colleagues, the overall culture of the midwives' workplace meant they had enough organisational support to facilitate women's alternative birth choices with relative ease. As such, they worked within enabling environments characterised by compassionate, collective leadership whereby an interplay between the midwives' personal motivations, and obstetric, managerial, institutional and effective leadership support was aligned (Maassen et al., 2021; RCPSYCH, 2020; West et al., 2017). The alignment fostered a culture in which women's alternative decisions were 'normalised', as Caz stated:

'This [supporting alternative birth choices] happens on a daily basis – it is not an unusual occurrence'.

James highlighted this interplay of an enabling environment during the creation of a new birth choices clinic to support women's alternative choices. While supporting women's choices was already embedded within the organisational culture, the new clinic was a proactive response to the statutory changes in supervision[5]. The overall achievements were highlighted as he jokingly referred to as *'being victims of our own success'*. This success was attributed to the local women asserting their agency and being steadfast in their decision-making to create a power transposition counter to the usual power imbalance between health professionals/organisations and service users. James shared the *'shock'* of new members of staff regarding the nature and scope of support for women's decisions, but how quickly they, the maternity professionals, *'fall into line'* reconstructing the power dynamic as one in women's favour (Begley et al., 2019):

yes they [the medics] are [supportive], I think partly because they are used to our women, new ones get a bit of a shock (laughs) when they come here because our women will say 'no I'm not doing it', they are quite vocal and our MSLC,[6] the consultants are really involved with, are extremely vocal and extremely passionate about tailoring the care to what women want, to what our population of women want and they've had to, for want of a better word, they've had to fall in line because you know it just causes them more stress than it does the women, because the women are quite formidable when they want to be, they'll just say 'no I'm not doing it' and we are quite lucky that a lot of our new consultants are quite young and dynamic and will just you know, they appreciate the women do have a choice.

Claire also conveyed non-hierarchical working relationships between midwives, doctors and management all supportive of women's choices. In part, Claire characterised this by the doctors knowing the midwives will support the women *'regardless'*, so a sense of positive defeatism fostered a supportive dynamic:

> … the two consultants who come out to our area to cover it have been there for quite a while and they kind of know that we will support the women regardless so they may as well go along with us.

Moreover, this was deemed a mutually beneficial arrangement for both the midwives and obstetricians due to an alignment of values and philosophies about maternity care. Such an alignment co-created and reinforced positive, respectful professional relationships. For example, women categorised with 'moderate risk' remained under midwifery-led care (counter to other organisations which would expect consultant-led care). This had two benefits. First, the midwives were able to directly support women with risk factors by making alternative birthing decisions in the knowledge they were supported by the multidisciplinary team. Second, the doctors were reported to value their time freed up to focus on *'women that really needed their input'*. The inference was, 'low-high risk' categories were applied judiciously to the satisfaction of both professional groups and birthing women and people in their care. Thus, enhancing the interprofessional working and overall psychological safety of the team:

> … quite often some are technically high risk but not that high risk, they don't even see them, they just sign them off, you know if we've got a lady with a slightly high BMI they'll just say 'a GTT [glucose tolerance test] at 28 weeks if ok MLC [midwife-led care]'… and they've got the time to use with the women who actually need their input so it works both ways.
>
> *[Claire]*

For context, Claire worked in an isolated rural area, a contributing factor of the cohesive relationships between midwives and doctors, and the acceptance of women's choices – a 'pragmatic' response to the realities of rural working. Similarly, Anna also worked rurally, where travelling time was factored into women's decision-making and contributed to a wider acceptance (doctors, management, organisation) of women having homebirths with risk factors. That the community midwives lived locally to the women and carried small caseloads (30–35 women p.a.) meant they were able to consistently offer intrapartum care. Attending the women was viewed as a safer alternative to the women travelling long distances, despite their risk factors. As such, a pragmatic approach to delivering maternity services contributed to the normalisation of women's choices, and cohesive working relationships which benefitted the psychological safety of the midwives working to support women's choices:

> Well, I work in X (place) it is very rural, it is sparsely populated, we don't have a district hospital at all, we only have birth centres … obviously we probably

get more women uhm say they would like to stay with us than you might get somewhere there is a hospital, just because they don't want to do that travel, actually a lot of them live well over an hour away from the hospital, and quite a long journey and if it's their third or fourth baby then it's a long way for them to go. For us, it is quite easy and that is probably just because we have small caseloads and geographically how we are placed, and the population we look after, yea, it makes it quite easy for us to do that sort of care really.

Stories of togetherness

Building on this idea of normalised practice, some of the emotion-stories were viewed within a sense of 'togetherness' within the midwives' team relationships. These relationships were characterised by closeness, friendship and mutual understanding – I refer to this as 'relational team working'. Such relational team working was expressed as inherently meaningful, as a source of joy and resilience and enhanced feelings of belonging (King's Fund, 2020). Strong team cohesiveness provided strength, safe learning environments and support, illustrating the King's Fund (2020) premises of what midwives need for staff engagement, wellbeing and flourishing. Moreover, different to those midwives in strong immediate teams but within wider toxic workplaces (discussed in Chapter 4 pg 79–80), these midwives worked in wider enabling and positive working environments (RCPSYCH, 2020). As such, working within both supportive immediate *and* wider teams facilitated joyful experiences and reciprocal gains with the women and other members of staff. For Kerry working in a close-knit team, she described the joy and the reciprocal gains when working closely with women in a caseloading model of care. Moreover, Kerry vividly and emotionally described the joy of working within an '*amazing*' team:

> … I had the best introduction to midwifery post-qualifying. I moved from a small cottage hospital to a large London trust to get experience but also to take up the opportunity to work as a caseload midwife. I joined a team of 5 amazing midwives who all took me under their wing. I also learnt so much from the women I had the privilege of getting to know throughout their varied pregnancy journeys … this team of midwives who are now like my sisters (laughs) they're just like yea I get emotional just thinking about it, they're just really really supportive and caring and I was able to ask questions, I wasn't afraid to ask questions …

The positivity of working within a like-minded team was perceived to be conducive to positive woman-centred care, highlighted by their standing in the local community:

> … I think that we had a good reputation in our area like, I remember one of the church's invited our team to come for a special evening or

something, we had a lovely community aspect, we would picnic every year with the women, they'd come back with their 4, 5, 6-year-old children that we'd been at their birth I definitely feel that it was yea, a really special, I was so lucky, really really lucky.

[Kerry]

Also passionate about working with women and her particular team was Amy, a homebirth team leader who asserted her *'privilege to work with really incredible midwives'*. When discussing the cohesiveness of the team, Amy attributed this to the open, respectful communication and ongoing learning within the team embodying the essence of psychological safety as per Edmondson (1999):

> … like I said we run these skills sessions, we listen to each other, we learn from each other, and I'm really privileged to work with really incredible midwives, so that kind of information sharing, 'what would you do if?' but just respecting the knowledge of our elders (laughing) as they have had these situations, and so we can learn from it so I'm like 'ok if I am ever in that situation, that's what I would do.'

Moreover, Amy highlighted a sense of togetherness when describing being *'inundated with volunteers'* when seeking midwives to set up a rota for a woman wanting a homebirth with multiple risk factors – indicative of team cohesion with shared values and skillsets. For these midwives to volunteer to support a complex homebirth demonstrates the implicit psychological safety embedded throughout the team culture, able to show up in potential vulnerability and thus, safe for 'interpersonal risk taking' (Edmondson, 1999):

> … we are really lucky to have a lot of community midwives who a. are confident in their skill set and b. very much believe in women's right to choose, so when I said 'is anyone interested in coming on board to put up an on-call rota' uhm I had, I was inundated with volunteers, you know I wasn't begging people and everyone was happy like 'yea I'll do that night, or I'll do that night' …

The sense of togetherness, belonging and camaraderie echoed throughout Amy's narrative accounts where she cited many examples of the positive *'top-down'* support her team received from senior members of staff. For example, she described the consultant midwife as the *'most amazing one going'*, the supervisors as *'powerful'* and management as *'supportive'*. Importantly, the support was not lip-service, in Amy's example below she demonstrated that the senior managers were also 'hands-on':

> … our deputy head when we've had two homebirths going on at the same time, he on multiple occasions gone out to a homebirth himself you know? You know homebirth is very protected, it's very sacred.

That Amy felt so supported by the senior team shows that the sense of togetherness went beyond her immediate team. These examples highlight an organisational culture of psychological safety and woman-centredness. Strong compassionate leadership created the conditions for Amy to flourish in her role as a team leader, embedding the positive characteristics of compassionate leadership (West et al., 2017) to create virtuous circles (Downe, 2010) of psychological safety. This was evident when Amy shared the support structures that were put in place for new or nervous midwives:

> So for my preceptors, because we do have preceptors to come out to community, they always do their on calls with me, they will be the first on call and I'm the second, but they call me at the start so we attend in pairs and they are always, it might be they're always with me, or with another senior team …

Amy's account also reflected some midwives preferred not to work with women making alternative birthing choices. However, within her working context, there were enough like-minded members of staff, women and midwives were able to get their needs met. Therefore, as a learning point to other organisations, what is needed to work this way is a 'critical mass' of maternity staff prepared, enabled and supported to fully operationalise woman-centred care, while also being respectful of the staff where alternative physiological births are too far outside of their comfort zone.

Stories of the sublime

These emotion stories captured and expressed feelings of warmth, love and compassion that permeated across five interviews. Moving accounts of love, awe, reverence, attunement, and tenderness were revealed – both towards the women in their care, and about birth itself. Embedded within the accounts was the notion of reciprocity, where the midwives received many emotional gains from their relationships with the women. Moreover, for one midwife, these exchanges occurred in a non-continuity model of care, thus offering an understanding of relational care within a fragmented model. That these accounts centred on the mother-midwife relationship with little expressed around their workplaces, was indicative of psychologically safe, enabling work environments (Maassen et al., 2021; RCPSYCH, 2020). The midwives' accounts were permeated with moments and experiences of joy which had profound meaning and long-lasting personal impacts. Such moments or experiences of joy are a substantial source of resilience (Brown, 2012) and these insights reveal what is possible, even within institutional working.

Jane provided a moving account in which she expressed reverence for the longstanding relationship she had with a couple throughout several pregnancies and births (sadly including a neonatal death). During her account of the woman's last birth, the depth of detail Jane remembered was striking. Through re-telling her story, Jane re-lived the moment; *'choking up'* which she reported as the *'pinnacle of her career'*. Throughout the interview, Jane voiced a strong sense of *'emotional attachment'* towards this family, which was conveyed in a heartfelt compulsion to do everything she could to make this birth the *'most positive experience that they could'*. She spoke of all the possibilities that could have occurred during the birth and finished each statement with *'I'll make it the best I can'*. My lasting impression was the profound impact this family had on Jane, walking alongside them throughout both joyful and sad times, they left a significant mark on Jane's heart. The following extract reveals the scope of the impact and the power of the connection between Jane and the couple. Moreover, coincidentally Jane bumped into the parents during the recruitment phase, whereby she had the opportunity to discuss the study with them and re-live together the specialness of the birth:

> one very frosty March morning I was called X [woman's name] husband and uhm, we, had a nice wood burning stove, ice cold marmalade on toast and she had a waterbirth and prior to her going into the pool, her little son had been in the pool so we made it quite jolly, and uhm then she birthed and she had little girl called X [name], it was one of the most privileged times that I have ever had in my career (choking up), it makes me want to cry when I think about it, because I felt privileged to be there, and to be part uh of their experience and you know I had been part of their life, and, for such a long time, you know because I had been through a lot with them. And when I had seen your flyer the other day, I actually met this couple shopping and I haven't seen them for several years and I said funny thing is, I was thinking about X [baby name] and how old she was now and I was saying to them how privileged I felt about being there, and they said uhm to me 'no, it was privilege that you were there with us, because you had been through so much with us', but like I said, it sounds silly, but it does make me want to cry because I do feel it was so, was one of the pinnacles of my career, it is something I will always think about, that that, that moment she came up in the water and it wouldn't have mattered if it had been another boy but I just thought the fact that it was a little girl (choking up) after that time [baby loss], that was fantastic as well.

Kelly also highlighted a longstanding connection between her and a couple when they requested her personally during two subsequent pregnancies which Kelly felt signalled *'trust'* between them. Such trust was deemed particularly relevant considering the woman's history whereby the woman was reported to have considerable fears of hospitals and clinical procedures which meant that throughout several pregnancies she had declined all screening/blood/urine tests and scans. Throughout Kelly's lengthy self-written narrative, she detailed many aspects of her care which I interpreted as a loving tenderness. Her words and actions denoted kindness and gentleness towards the woman, demonstrating respect for her choices throughout the narrative. Kelly relayed purposefully seeking the woman's trust through deliberate actions; seeking permission to personally care for the woman (who was out of her usual catchment), and responsive care when the woman became distressed, visiting the family every two weeks[7] and taking an interest in the other children as a way to *'encourage her to talk and be confident in trusting that her choices would be respected'* and *'going on call'* for the birth. As the pregnancy progressed, Kelly appeared to foster a sense of protectiveness towards the woman, symbolising the connection she felt. The following extract highlights a combination of Kelly's protectiveness, connection and responsive care:

> I arranged a meeting at their home with myself and the supervisor. I felt it was really important for me to be there to support X [couple]. The supervisor explained the risks of having a baby at home and asked whether she would consent to a presentation scan. X [name] became tearful at this suggestion and the supervisor did not press the issue. It was agreed at this meeting that I would be on-call for her which I was very happy to do. I felt it was much more likely that she would call me to attend the birth this time rather than leave it too late as she did last time.

Kelly's actions and experiences of providing compassionate care can be contextualised by her midwifery philosophy which is underpinned by two significant beliefs. First, she believed birth to have *'massively long-lasting effects'* throughout a woman's life, so the mother-midwife relationship is *'hugely important'*. Second, she believed the core components of safe and satisfying care were *'appropriate antenatal care and a trusting relationship'*. Most striking was the reciprocal nature of the trusting relationship, in which Kelly reported a *'relationship of trust enables me to feel safe when supporting women who make choices outside the normal'*. Therefore, highlights how feelings of safety work both ways within the mother-midwife relationship – also identified in Chapter 3.

Susan also conveyed the value of connection and trust in a midwife-woman relationship for any birthing choice, including those deemed outside of the guidelines. Her account was characterised by a sense of attunement where she employed deliberate actions to harmonise with a woman in labour. While Susan worked in a fragmented model of care, she explained how she worked to achieve a space in which the women felt they were the centre of their experience, and how much they mattered. When I asked her how she achieved this, she responded with vivid language suggesting simple acts of kindness foster mother-midwife attunement:

> You just, you just talk nicely to people and you go to that place where they are rather than expecting them to somehow meet you on your plane, it's theirs, it's their space it's their experience and you go to where they are or and if they're not in a place that is conducive for labour cos they're in a heightened state of anxiety or feeling they have to be very talky to make me feel comfortable cos they're meeting a new person or they're in a strange environment you go in and you put yourself in that space, you talk softer

and and you respond less, you respond to make them feel comfortable so if they are very talky you might be slightly more talky at the beginning but consciously talking less and less to uh and being ok with silence so they get that feeling without you saying 'it's ok not to talk now' [loud] (laughs) that they get that sense that this is ok, this is about them, you make it all about them and because the place where labour happens best.

Moreover, during the interview, Susan reflected upon the evolution of her (longstanding) midwifery practice. It was during a massage research study she witnessed a different style of midwifery practice which *'triggered a change'* both within her professional practice and also personally. Susan constructed this pivotal moment as a time for *'personal growth'* kindling a spiritual self. Within this context, Susan's workplace environment and interrelationships created an enabling, learning space where personal and professional growth was fostered – meeting and elevating her core needs to where flourishing could occur (King's Fund, 2020). Moreover, Susan perceived a mutual benefit in her new style of caregiving, where she gained *'more'* and gained a stronger reverence of birth and the power held by those women birthing:

> yea that was so lovely it was uhm really wonderful being in that room uhm and quite eye opening to the power of just silence, watching and it was lovely, it was really lovely [observing the research midwife conduct massage on someone during labour]. So that you know triggered a change and then I think personal growth away from being a midwife kind of finding mindfulness and meditations getting to know myself more deeply, more spiritually... being present with women is uhm is I guess is a two way street whatever me being present for them, it has brought more for me being able to watch that whole energetic dance you know the whole fear thing and seeing, you get to see uh life, the microcosm of life itself the entirety of your existence played out in a myriad of ways by different people in this dance of labour that sort of you know, the women who say no to it and fight it and uh are fearful you see how that works or the ones who say yes to it, sink in to it, and go with the flow of it and you see how that works and all the different and all the different types of ways along that spectrum.

Meeting the needs of midwives, meeting the needs of women

This chapter has shown how psychologically safe workplace environments meet a fundamental need of midwives (King's Fund, 2020). An alignment between the values of the midwives and the institutions toward woman-centredness cultivated an enabling environment for the midwives to deliver alternative physiological birth care. Characterised by trust and respect with embedded support across the hierarchical structures and positive workplaces created the conditions for midwives to find fulfilment in their roles. Such positive impact harnessed by consistently working within their values, a sense of belonging and crucially, meaningful contribution, are fundamental components of workforce sustainability (Crowther et al., 2016; King's Fund, 2020). In stark contrast to Chapter 4, in these accounts, the emphasis of the story's changed – a de-centring of their workplaces, secured by psychological safety, created the space to bring the women's birth stories to the fore. Unburdened by conflict, a lessened mental and emotional load allowed the midwives to not only get on with the job but to flourish; experiencing joy through relational care that offered reciprocal gains, meaning-making and personal affect. These experiences of joy, awe and wonder are a source of resilience and likely contributing factors to why midwives stay (Sullivan et al., 2011). Through gathering these insights, the findings conveyed how an organisation can shift from the oppressive cultures we observed in Chapter 4 toward one of greater woman-centredness. In the next chapter, we revisit Chapters 3–5 within a new lens, a new way of looking at this data – 'Stigmatised to normalised practice' offers a theoretical model to explain the findings revealed so far.

Notes

1 Also see (Catling et al., 2017; Crowther et al., 2016; Sullivan et al., 2011).
2 As the midwives in this storyline were in leadership positions, mostly their role was to develop the complex care plans and provide support to the staff delivering the care. In this section, I refer to midwife caregivers as those delivering the care plans and who were unlikely to be involved in the care planning discussions, which at times is a source of tension.
3 Women who have experienced stillbirth.
4 Human factors is a concept frequently associated with the aviation industry, which saw radical safety improvements as they worked with this conceptual approach. Primarily, it removes a blame culture and fosters an open learning culture, where mistakes/poor outcomes are a collective responsibility rather than just an individual (Ansari et al., 2020; Boston-Fleischhauer, 2008).
5 As discussed in Chapter 1, in 2017, legislative changes removed statutory supervision for midwives. Supervision had historically been used in many areas as a mechanism of support for women and midwives who make alternative birthing decisions. A new model has since been introduced but organisations are not legally obliged to implement it, therefore, some areas are now lacking an equivalent service (DH, 2017; Parliamentary and Health Service Ombudsman, 2013).
6 Maternity Services Liaison Committee which comprises of lay members, multi-professionals coming together to improve local maternity services, now reformed as 'Maternity Voices Partnership' (NMP, 2022).
7 Two weekly visits throughout a pregnancy are not the usual pattern of care and is above and beyond most NHS midwifery services.

References

Ansari, S. P., Rayfield, M. E., Wallis, V. A., Jardine, J. E., Morris, E. P., & Prosser-Snelling, E. (2020). A safety evaluation of the impact of maternity-orientated human factors training on safety culture in a tertiary maternity unit. *Journal of Patient Safety*, 16(4), e359–e366.

Begley, K., Daly, D., Panda, S., & Begley, C. (2019). Shared decision-making in maternity care: Acknowledging and overcoming epistemic defeaters. *Journal of Evaluation in Clinical Practice*, 25(6), 1113–1120. doi: 10.1111/jep.13243

Boston-Fleischhauer, C. (2008). Enhancing healthcare process design with human factors engineering and reliability science, part 1: Setting the context. *JONA: The Journal of Nursing Administration*, 38(1), 27–32.

Brown, B. (2012). *Daring Greatly: How the Courage to Be Vulnerable Transforms the Way We Live, Love, Parent, and Lead*. Gotham.

Brown, B. (2018). *Dare to Lead: Brave Work. Tough Conversations. Whole Hearts*. Vermilion.

Catling, C. J., Reid, F., & Hunter, B. (2017). Australian midwives' experiences of their workplace culture. *Women Birth*, 30(2), 137–145. doi: 10.1016/j.wombi.2016.10.001

Crowther, S., Hunter, B., McAra-Couper, J., Warren, L., Gilkison, A., Hunter, M., Fielder, A., & Kirkham, M. (2016). Sustainability and resilience in midwifery: A discussion paper. *Midwifery*, 40, 40–48. doi: 10.1016/j.midw.2016.06.005

DH. (2017). *The Nursing and Midwifery Council – Amendments to Modernise Midwifery Regulation and Improve the Effectiveness and Efficiency of Fitness to Practise Processes Consultation Report*. Leeds: Department of Health. https://assets.publishing.service.gov.uk/government/uploads/system/uploads/attachment_data/file/582494/Consultation_report.pdf

Downe, S. (2010). Beyond evidence-based medicine: Complexity and stories of maternity care. *Journal of Evaluation in Clinical Practice*, 16(1), 232–237. doi: 10.1111/j.1365–2753.2009.01357.x

Edmondson, A. (1999). Psychological safety and learning behavior in work teams. *Administrative Science Quarterly*, 44(2), 350–383. doi: 10.2307/2666999

Edmondson, A., & Harvey, J. (2017). *Extreme Teaming: Lessons in Complex, Cross-Sector Leadership*. Emerald Group Publishing Limited.

Hunter, B. (2010). Mapping the emotional terrain of midwifery: What can we see and what lies ahead? *International Journal of Work Organisation and Emotion*, 3(3), 253–269.

Hunter, B., Henley, J., Fenwick, J., Sidebotham, M., & Pallant, J. (2018). *Work, Health and Emotional Lives of Midwives in the United Kingdom: The UK WHELM Study*. Cardiff: Cardiff University. https://www.rcm.org.uk/media/2924/work-health-and-emotional-lives-of-midwives-in-the-united-kingdom-the-uk-whelm-study.pdf

King's Fund. (2020). *The Courage of Compassion: Supporting Nurses and Midwives to Deliver High-Quality Care*. London: King's Fund. https://www.kingsfund.org.uk/sites/default/files/2020-09/The%20courage%20of%20compassion%20full%20report_0.pdf

Maassen, S. M., van Oostveen, C., Vermeulen, H., & Weggelaar, A. M. (2021). Defining a positive work environment for hospital healthcare professionals: A Delphi study. *PloS One*, 16(2), e0247530. doi: 10.1371/journal.pone.0247530

Nembhard, I. M., & Edmondson, A. C. (2006). Making it safe: The effects of leader inclusiveness and professional status on psychological safety and improvement efforts in health care teams. *Journal of Organizational Behavior*, 27(7), 941–966. doi: 10.1002/job.413

NMP. (2022). *National Maternity Voices*. https://nationalmaternityvoices.org.uk/

O'Donovan, R., & McAuliffe, E. (2020). Exploring psychological safety in healthcare teams to inform the development of interventions: Combining observational, survey and interview data. *BMC Health Services Research*, 20(1), 810. doi: 10.1186/s12913-020-05646-z

Parliamentary and Health Service Ombudsman. (2013). Midwifery supervision and regulation: Recommendations for change. Unite: The Stationery Office Limited. https://www.ombudsman.org.uk/

RCM. (2016). *Why Midwives Leave Revisited.* London: RCM. https://www.proquest.com/openview/914f52ff00a17d34da28f892b2d4985d/1.pdf?pq-origsite=gscholar&cbl=506295https

RCPSYCH. (2020). *Ten Evidence-Based Reasons for Embedding Values-Based 'Enabling Environments' in Health Care.* London: Royal College of Psychiatrists. https://www.rcpsych.ac.uk/docs/default-source/improving-care/ccqi/quality-networks/enabling-environments-ee/enabling-environments-in-health-care-10-reasons.pdf?sfvrsn=996c3058_4

Renfrew, M., McFadden, A., Bastos, M., Campbell, J., Channon, A., Cheung, N., Silva, D., Downe, S., Kennedy, H., Malata, A., McCormick, F., Wick, L., & Declercq, E. (2014). Midwifery and quality care: Findings from a new evidence-informed framework for maternal and newborn care. *Lancet*, 384(9948), 1129–1145. doi: 10.1016/S0140–6736(14)60789-3

Robertson, J. H., & Thomson, A. M. (2016). An exploration of the effects of clinical negligence litigation on the practice of midwives in England: A phenomenological study. *Midwifery*, 33, 55–63. doi: 10.1016/j.midw.2015.10.005

Sullivan, K., Lock, L., & Homer, C. S. E. (2011). Factors that contribute to midwives staying in midwifery: A study in one area health service in New South Wales, Australia. *Midwifery*, 27(3), 331–335. doi: 10.1016/j.midw.2011.01.007

Walsh, D. (2007). *Improving Maternity Services: Small Is Beautiful - Lessons from a Birth Centre.* Radcliffe Publishing.

West, M., & Bailey, S. (2019). *Five Myths of Compassionate Leadership.* https://www.kingsfund.org.uk/blog/2019/05/five-myths-compassionate-leadership

West, M., Collins, B., Eckhert, R., & Chowla, R. (2017). *Caring to Change: How Compassionate Leadership Can Stimulate Innovation in Health Care.* London: The King's Fund. https://www.kingsfund.org.uk/publications/caring-change

West, M., Eckert, R., Steward, K., & Pamore, B. (2014). *Developing Collective Leadership for Health Care.* London: King's Fund. https://www.kingsfund.org.uk/sites/default/files/field/field_publication_file/developing-collective-leadership-kingsfund-may14.pdf

6

STIGMATISED TO NORMALISED PRACTICE

A new lens

So far, Chapters 3–5 illuminated the study participants' experiences of facilitating alternative physiological births, sharing insights into how they delivered care and the polarised spectrum of their workplace environments. While this study only included the perspectives of the midwives, their insights resonated with wider literature and contributed to the further understanding of the realities of everyday midwifery practice. In this chapter, the evidence from Chapters 3–5 is advanced further using theory to explore and explain the sociocultural-political influences on the midwives' practice. All the findings were reanalysed using theories of stigma/normal, and deviance/positive deviance to situate the midwives' practice within their micro, meso and macro working contexts, culminating in a six-domain theoretical model (see Appendix 3). This third analysis placed the midwives on a spectrum of 'stigmatised-normalised practice' synthesising and explaining their experiences within their immediate teams, wider teams and more broadly, their organisational culture. Therefore, this chapter reframes the study findings to provide a deepened understanding of the midwives' practice of delivering alternative physiological birth care; through which lessons can be learned to facilitate wider improvements. First, an overview of the theories used is presented, followed by an exploration of the six domains within the theoretical model.

Normal/stigma, deviance/positive deviance

Stigma can only be understood in relation to constructs of 'normalcy' and vice versa – to be stigmatised correlates with perceptions of being 'abnormal' (Misztal, 2001). 'Normalcy' is a social construct located within particular social, cultural and historical meanings (Frost, 2011). Misztal (2001) argued that notions of 'normal' manifest as the 'taken-for-granted' value of everyday life. A sense of

DOI: 10.4324/9781003265443-6

normality makes the world predictable and reliable – fostering a sense of 'things as usual' (Misztal, 2001). Goffman (1963) viewed normality as a collective representation (of a given group/society) sustained by interactional rituals. Thus, notions of normalcy are based on implicit and explicit social interactions where people gradually acquire practical and tacit knowledge socialising them to act in a particular way in a particular environment (Goffman, 1963). Therefore, normalcy operates within relational contexts, contributing to social order, with both positive and negative consequences. If a sense of normality fosters feelings of predictability and reliability, Misztal (1996) suggests its outcome is social trust and furthers cooperation through reinforced expectations of reciprocity. Sabel (1993) defined trust as '*the mutual confidence that no party to an exchange will exploit another's vulnerability (p.1133)*'. Therefore, risk and uncertainty are features of mutual trust (Sheppard & Sherman, 1998). Conversely, Garfinkel (1963), considers it is trust first, which constructs the sense of normality and by consequence creates social order. Perhaps, trust is involved in both the production of and a consequence of normality and regardless of whether trust is a component or a product of retaining a sense of normality, social trust can be seen as a 'stabilizer of social order' (Misztal, 2001, p. 313). In this context, notions of normalcy are tied to notions of trust, cooperation and reciprocity (Luhmann, 2000; Scott, 1999).

Goffman (1971) provided a theoretical lens to examine social interactions to discern how normal order is constructed, including 'normal appearances', asserting the appearance of normality[1] counted more than actually *being* normal. Such appearances of normality limit the perceptions of threats to those around us, enhancing peaceful, safe environments (Misztal, 2001). The preservation of daily routines, and ordinary living, means the reality of unpredictability is concealed (Misztal, 2001). For individuals whose beliefs and attitudes are not aligned with the social order, this can require effort for them to 'pass as normal' (Misztal, 2001; Frost, 2011). 'Passing as normal' is argued to be bound in conceptualisations of morality, therefore, being perceived as abnormal, or causing disruptive events to others' perceptions of normalcy can lead to moral judgements about the individual (Garfinkel, 1963). Such acts may be viewed as 'deviant' which relates to attributes, attitudes, behaviour or actions perceived to violate local norms (Adler & Adler, 2015; Dodge, 1985). To be perceived as 'abnormal' or 'deviant' gives rise to stigma – defined by Goffman (1963) as a personal attribute '*that can be deeply discrediting, which reduces the whole persons to tainted and discounted others (p.3)*', whereas Herek (2009) later defined stigma within a societal lens:

> the negative regard, inferior status and relative powerlessness that society collectively accords to people who possess a particular characteristic or belong to a particular group or category. (p. 441)

Frost (2011) argued this shift in definition moved the origin of stigma from an individual identity (perceived defect) to a societal level whereby meanings attributed to deviancy behaviours and stigma are socially, culturally and historically located, and can change over time (Frost, 2011; Herek, 2009). Link and Phelan (2001) highlighted components of stigma as: labelling, stereotyping, separation, status loss and discrimination. Their model argues that labelled/stereotyped people are placed in distinct categories, thus 'separated' – accounting for divisions of 'us and them' (Link & Phelan, 2001). Notions of us and them can be traced back to Émile Durkheim's [1912] (1995) seminal work recognising the power of shared group identification. Durkheim claimed shared experiences, values, norms and beliefs contribute to feelings of belonging and solidarity and reinforce group identification (Durkheim, 1995). Danger occurs when a group perceives a threat to their stability by 'others' (Beyer et al., 2014), which creates the conditions for labelling and stigmatisation to mitigate against the threat (Beyer et al., 2014). Moreover, the process of stigmatising 'others' may strengthen the social bonds of those who are in the 'in' group (Durkheim, 1995).

Power imbalances are also a characteristic of stigmatisation (Foucault, 1975; Link & Phelan, 2001). Foucault (1975) argued institutional hierarchies enforce 'normalisation' via disciplinary tactics to create and retain power and maintain social norms. Hierarchies play a significant role in power differentials, arising in small informal social groups and macro groups i.e., institutions (Link & Phelan, 2001). Where a person is situated within a hierarchy is largely dependent upon their perceived status where for some people, they may experience low status from the outset of joining an organisation, often related to discrimination i.e., gender, ethnicity, class, and job role (Link & Phelan, 2001). Others may experience a loss of status occurring by a process of devaluation, discrimination and prejudice (Link & Phelan, 2001). Low status and/or a lowering of status can have negative consequences for the individual mentally, emotionally, physically and financially (Phelan et al., 2008).

Recent research has identified experiences of stigma operate as a 'social stressor' which leads to individuals trying to adapt intrapersonally and/or interpersonally often with negative consequences (Frost, 2011).[2] The onus may be placed upon the stigmatised person to manage others' perceptions of them, known as 'stigma management' (Frost, 2011). This form of 'management' mirrors Goffman's (1963) 'passing as normal' whereby a stigmatised person has to decide whether to conceal or make visible their stigma[3]. Whilst concealing one's stigma can be a protective mechanism, it is also a cognitive burden (Frost, 2011). In addition, internalising stigma can impact one's self-identity resulting in self-devaluation (Meyer, 2003), causing several negative impacts on a person's mental and physical health including cardiovascular disease, increased risk behaviours, poor job performance and satisfaction (Frost, 2011).

Frost (2011) also identified coping mechanisms stigmatised people may use; positive strategies include meditation, expressive writing or attempting to change the circumstances (Thoits, 1995).[4] Conversely, maladaptive coping strategies such as increased alcohol, drug, smoking, or food consumption may be used at a cost to physical health (Hayward et al., 2018).[5] Group-level coping processes include the reliance on others in a stigmatised group to provide physical and psychologically safe environments, with some evidence to suggest it can reduce the negative ill effects of being stigmatised (Meyer, 2003).[6] Other researchers have highlighted how some people employ meaning-making processes and narrative strategies to overcome the delimiting effects of stigmatisation (Crocker & Major, 1989; Shih, 2004). Unger (1998) a critical feminist, argued 'positive marginality' may foster agency and resilience, an alternative response for individuals with stigma stressors. Active resistance and the assertion of agency to reclaim experiences of being marginalised can manifest as activism and attempts at social change (Campbell & Deacon, 2006).[7]

Positive marginality can also be viewed within the lens of positive deviance. Spreitzer and Sonenshein (2003) defined positive deviancy as the intentional behaviours departing from the norms of a referent group in honourable ways. Positive deviants tend to be those (individuals or whole teams) with innovative strategies and demonstrate high performance in a given area (Bradley et al., 2009). In a conceptual review of positive deviancy, Herington & van de Fliert (2018) consider positive deviancy to be a theoretical concept or a practical strategy. From a theoretical perspective, positive deviancy can aid understanding of how and why positive deviancy occurs, and the circumstances under which it occurs, thereby contributing knowledge regarding human social processes. From a practical perspective, studying positive deviancy offers the development of frameworks to facilitate the improvements of social problems (Herington & van de Fliert, 2018).[8] Singhal and Dura (2017) argued that increased attention to positive deviancy signalled a 'practice turn' in social science studies – moving away from an evidence-based practice approach where problems were researched, disseminated and decontextualised from everyday practice, to 'practice-based evidence' which is a practical problem-solving, bottom-up approach e.g., this study.

'Stigmatised to normalised practice' – A theoretical model

Weaving these opposing theories through the data, the spectrum of experience reported in Chapters 3–5 can be observed and accounted for as 'stigmatised to normalised practice' (see Figure 6.1). However, these conceptions are socially and culturally contingent; what might be deemed deviant behaviour in one context, may be normal elsewhere or vice versa. Therefore, it is important to acknowledge the specific cultural context of this theoretical model as relating to the experiences of NHS midwives' willingly facilitative of alternative physiological births within their particular workplace environments at the time of the study.

Stigmatised practice

This domain represents three midwives whose normal midwifery practice was to facilitate women's choices but who were isolated, marginalised and experienced negative reprisals. As described in Chapter 4, these included investigations and referrals to the professional Nursing and Midwifery Council for unsafe

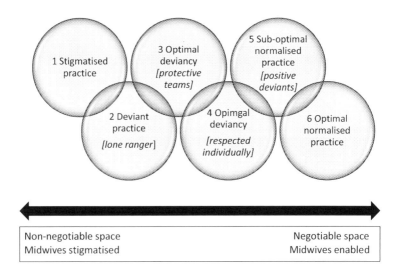

FIGURE 6.1   Theoretical model: stigmatised to normalised practice

practices (all of whom eventually were found to have no case to answer). In this domain, the midwives appeared to be situated completely outside of local socio-cultural working norms and were perceived negatively, as 'deviants' (Dodge, 1985). This resulted in varying degrees of stigmatisation. In two instances, poor birth outcomes made 'visible' the midwives' 'deviant' practice. In the other instance, Beatrice's deviance was noticed when she discussed her planned clinical care with an obstetrician which alerted her team as not complying with the social norms. As highlighted in Chapter 4 Beatrice was caring for a woman with gestational diabetes opting for intermittent auscultation of the fetal heart rate and the birth pool rather than continuous electronic fetal monitoring (on land) as recommended in the local guidelines. Such a care plan was not deemed culturally acceptable and despite no adverse outcome, Beatrice's 'deviance' catalysed a chain reaction of events culminating in supervised practice (highlighted in Chapter 4):

> I mooched into the office not thinking a great deal of it and the office is always full, they have the consultant in there with a registrar … I have worked for this guy before, and to me he is probably one of the most inoffensive courteous guy you could imagine… this time [after sharing the care plan] I got a look like I was something on the bottom of his shoe and practically saying I was leading her down the path to obstetric disaster … and of course this exchange is taking place in front of at least another four people with the door of the office open …

In all three examples, not working within the guidelines was problematic within their workplace context. Guidelines can be seen as a cultural representation of patriarchal and hierarchical dominance (Berg, 2000)[9] and a tool of '*disciplinary power*' (Foucault, 1975). Drawing on Misztal's (1996) notions of normalcy which fosters predictability, reliability and a 'sense of things as usual' then these midwives appeared to cause tension and threatened the 'social order' of stability. As such, they were 'othered' for not sustaining the expected cultural 'interactional rituals' of working within guidelines (Goffman, 1963). The disruption of social order was particularly profound in situations where a poor outcome occurred. The public nature of the reprisals or investigations after an adverse event meant they were no longer able to 'pass as normal' (Goffman, 1963). Separation as a 'disciplinary tactic' (Foucault, 1975) occurred via either removing the midwife from her clinical area, stopping a service the midwife was leading or through prolonged investigations (see Chapter 4). Such separation and the stigma associated with being investigated resulted in status loss and discrimination (Link & Phelan, 2001) rendering the midwives powerless until the investigations had been completed:

> I don't think I will ever recover from it, it has coloured the rest of my life forever, the ongoing effects were absolutely massive. I was suicidal … it took 14 months for the [supervised] practice to be signed off. I was isolated from the ward, I was sent down to work in the antenatal clinic. I had to give up working with an agency … caused a great deal of financial hardship …
>
> *(Beatrice)*

Moreover, these midwives felt they were judged to be immoral due to violating local social norms (Garfinkel, 1963) – 'discredited' via negative labelling which included direct accusations of 'brainwashing' women into making choices outside of the guidelines (Goffman, 1963). Such 'discrediting' by their wider teams through the perception of being 'dangerous' midwives resulted in their stigmatised position and greater scrutiny. Moreover, constructs of 'bad choices' or 'bad midwives' belie a misogynistic social norm of assumed compliance of midwives and women (Rock, 2007), as highlighted by Georgina:

> … but again the underlying doubt is always is this 'is it actually her choice?' or has the midwife convinced her to have a physiological third stage because the midwife would always choose what is natural' and that is disturbing to me because uhm it belies the notion that actually women choose what you need them to choose and that's the way perhaps other health professionals operate, whereas you know whereas people don't notice when women under my care choose to have an epidural or choose an active third stage they just always notice when they choose not to.

Negative consequences of being stigmatised were found across all three accounts including the deterioration of the midwives' mental, emotional and physical wellbeing (Frost, 2011). The midwives' financial wellbeing was also negatively impacted due to limitations placed on their opportunities to practice. The midwives adapted to these experiences in different ways. One left the organisation and sought support for her midwifery practice elsewhere. Another midwife reported making significant changes to her midwifery practice resulting in 'defensive practice' (Ortashi et al., 2013) by avoiding working alone during intrapartum clinical care and making plans to leave the profession. Beatrice sought a research role by way of 'active resistance' (Campbell & Deacon, 2006):

> Could I leave midwifery? ... It is better to build bridges than walls. Or more prosaically, 'it is better to be inside pissing out, than outside pissing in'. So I am researching to a standard that might even attract the approbation of Don Quixote by achieving a marriage of facts and truth. And preparing for my next joust with a windmill.

Deviant practice [lone ranger]

This domain represented the eight midwives whose personal practice of facilitating women's choices was not within local norms of practice, where they worked in relative isolation with little support – a '*lone ranger*'. The midwives differed from those in the previous domain as they practised their preferred midwifery whilst retaining some membership of their teams. However, those relationships were characterised by frequent conflicts and a lack of support. The midwives felt identified as social 'deviants' (Dodge, 1985) which they managed by a combination of 'fighting' back, subversive tactics to deliver woman–centred care and attempts to 'pass as normal' (Goffman, 1963). The misalignment between the midwives' notions of 'normalcy' and their colleagues left the midwives vulnerable to the consequences of stigmatisation. Like the midwives in the previous domain, this misalignment led to moral distress (as seen in Chapter 4) and financial hardship as the midwives reduced their working hours to cope with the distress and/or required sick leave. However, the salient difference was the midwives in this domain did not experience being investigated, although, did voice fears of punitive action. Therefore, through a process of 'stigma management' (Goffman, 1963) the midwives '*picked their battles*' to maintain social working relationships, suggesting these midwives were unable to practice the full scope of midwifery all of the time:

> I think I have been lucky, I have been lucky because I just try to go under the radar really, it's no good to try and engage with them, they want you to get on and do it because it fulfils the need for the service, I cover the service needs and they are happy enough with that and the rest of it I just I suppose I am a bit resigned as to that's the way it is and I don't think it will be any different I don't think.

> *[Maria]*

While this was a source of distress, it meant the midwives attempted to manage the tensions arising from their practice by limiting 'threats to the social order' (Misztal, 1996). Such practices were arguably employed to garner trust, cooperation and reciprocity (Misztal, 2001) from their colleagues and to retain group membership. Ginny referred to it as *'playing the long game'* – picking her battles, keeping up appearances long enough to be in a job role with more power (i.e., senior midwife) in which she could actualise her midwifery ideal. Such acts of stigma management were suggestive of the power imbalances within the participant's workplace. In these situations, the onus appeared to be on the midwife to manage the tensions arising from others' perceptions of their midwifery practice whilst continuing to deliver what they felt to be authentic midwifery. As such, these midwives were in somewhat powerless positions, where fears of *'penalties'* for their midwifery practice created tensions:

> … the way that the maternity services are, where I work there is a fear that is very large it's a fear, yea it's something I am very very conscious of, there are things that I'd be thinking about, like documentation, how am I expressing what's happening, how do you justify yourself? To a probably negative critic …
>
> *[Meg]*

Furthermore, the midwives managed the tensions in practice to prevent escalation of their perceived 'deviancy' to the full extent of stigmatisation. Perceptions or experiences of 'surveillance' (Foucault, 1975) could be attributed to the midwives' awareness they needed to 'manage stigma' (Goffman, 1963). Foucault (1975) argued hierarchised, continuous and functional surveillance contributed to an integration of systemic power, both explicit as it is everywhere, yet insidious as it is largely silenced. This was highlighted by Alex:

> … but whereas you go onto an obstetric unit you do find that the doctors, although you are supposedly autonomous, they are watching over your care. The way the birth suite is set up where they have all the monitors and the computer IT systems when you are in the room with a lady and you write down everything but are being watched by the doctors at the same time …

Optimal deviancy [protective teams]

This domain represented the eight midwives whose personal practice of facilitating women's choices was normal within their immediate team but deemed 'deviant' in the wider organisational context. Therefore, 'optimal deviancy' conveys how they worked well within positive teams operating to deliver woman-centred care while also experiencing challenges elsewhere within their organisation – their way of working was reported as not supported by their wider organisational teams. However, unique to this domain, all the midwives were community-based which may have accounted for a particular sense of 'us and them' (Link & Phelan, 2001) between their immediate teams and their wider hospital-based teams. Operating within a 'relational model of working', the midwives' immediate co-workers were friends indicating closeness, mutual respect and reciprocity. Being able to rely on each other, bounce ideas, to provide support when work was challenging characterised the midwives' experiences. As such, the teams operated as a source of resilience, protecting individual vulnerability (see Chapter 4) and the threat of full stigmatisation.

Midwives in this domain worked within teams with 'like-minded' 'deviants'; where a woman-centred philosophy of care was mostly deliverable and was 'normalised practice'. The midwives who worked in this context shared the values and beliefs of the team, mutually reinforcing their team's social norms; reinforcing their sense of 'normalcy' to support alternative physiological birth choices, sustained by interactional rituals (Goffman 1963). This alignment created space for the midwives to acquire the practice and tacit knowledge to enact their preferred midwifery philosophy (Goffman, 1963):

> I think I just liked the way they worked I just knew that's what I definitely wanted to do … I think probably just working with the right people in the right team … I know very much that I don't work well in the hospital, I really like being at home so by virtue of that, you start working with people that feel the same and you start with women who feel really strongly about that as well, so it becomes a little bit more normal, and it snowballs from there.
>
> *[Rose]*

Midwives in this domain reported trust was constructed through an alignment of values and beliefs among their team members, which was continually mutually reinforcing (Garfinkel, 1963; Misztal, 2001). Thus, trust was constructed and perpetuated by the normalcy of delivering/practising woman-centred care, as highlighted by Laura:

> It is a real nice caseloading job which you don't really get in the normal community setting … But we all have the same ethos, and we all work really well together and I think that's what helps us, cos we have got really good [homebirth] rates as well and being a really tight knit team, and knowing exactly how each of us works helps us um, support each other… but I think when you are with people that support you and also that are there to have your back as well, it really makes a difference.

Furthermore, feelings of psychological safety were enhanced by reciprocal trust whereby they felt enabled to ask questions and not to fear ridicule (Edmondson,

1999). Whilst trust was central to the immediate team relationships, this did not transfer across to wider hospital teams. Divisions of 'us and them' as mentioned earlier were reported as being labelled negatively (Link & Phelan, 2001) as midwives with a *'reputation'*, or *'troublemakers'* or *'brainwashing women'* (highlighted in Chapter 4) – so far a consistent finding across perceptions of deviant midwifery. Contributing to the divisions between community and hospital midwives, are likely the different working practices or structures, roles and physical locations. By virtue of their role, community midwives often have greater independence than hospital midwives and are less visible on the wards. A lack of personal relationships between community midwives and those working in the hospital was felt to be caused by reduced opportunities to build intra-professional relationships:

> … and also being community midwives they don't know very much we probably get more suspicion than other people which is slightly off topic but they think 'who is this person in their own clothes who I have never met before, who has waltzed into labour ward in her sandals' or something (laughs).
>
> *[Rose]*

Optimal deviancy [respected individually]

This domain represented the four midwives who normally facilitated alternative women's choices but where such practices were not fully embedded across their immediate teams or wider organisational cultures. In contrast to the previous domain, where the midwives operated within 'protective teams', these midwives, were largely able to deliver woman–centred care without 'protective teams'. These midwives reported their colleagues typified their practice as 'different' but were not labelled or stereotyped as (morally) 'deviant'. Where conflicts or challenges arose, these did not appear to threaten their colleagues' notions of 'normalcy' (Misztal, 2001), in turn, the midwives in this domain did not appear to feel threatened by their colleagues. Overall, the midwives felt respected in their working environments as autonomous practitioners, and were largely able to deliver woman–centred care unencumbered. The midwives in this domain developed (largely) positive working relationships with their midwifery and multidisciplinary colleagues, despite their different midwifery styles. Although all the midwives in this domain reported several frustrations regarding their organisational cultures, these did not detrimentally affect their personal midwifery practice. They garnered the respect of their colleagues which essentially meant they were trusted to *'get on with it'*. This might be explained by their extensive clinical experience – all of them had over 20 year's clinical experience and/or had been employed within the organisation for many years. Conceivably, these factors are likely to have contributed to the development of respectful and trusting working relationships. Highlighting this, Catherine described conversations with obstetric colleagues

who were supportive of women's alternative decision-making, *if* Catherine was the midwife caregiver:
   '[in relation to supporting VBAC]

>   but I think some of the obstetricians from the conversations that we have, kind of think that midwives might not pick up on scar rupture and things if they've not got a CTG to rely on uhm but they come like 'you're expecting inexperienced midwives who perhaps don't have the same philosophy, to look after these women and will they actually pick it up?'… to me 'it will be fine if you're looking after them …'

Others referred to being identified as a *'type of midwife'* particularly suited to women requesting out of guidelines care. In these situations, rather than the midwife experiencing negative labelling (Link & Phelan, 2001), it was the women deemed 'deviant'. Therefore, the midwives practice was perceived as beneficial to the wider teams who did not want to care for women making alternative physiological birth choices. Therefore, what could be deemed deviant behaviour in other contexts, was viewed favourably in these specific situations:

>   The birth plan for this lady was quite extensive and had been discussed at length with the consultant midwife prior to coming in. At handover she was proclaimed as 'one for me', with rolled eyes at the birth plan …
>
>   *[Susan]*

Sub-optimal normalised practice [positive deviants]

This domain represented the eight midwives who facilitated women's choices as part of their usual practice. In addition, they were positive deviant's aka 'change agents' (Herington & van de Fliert, 2018). Working to improve women's access to choices and embed woman-centred care within their organisations, they were tasked with cultivating institutional cultural change. Unique to this domain, all midwives were in leadership (senior) positions and were 'positive deviants' by virtue of their role. They were enabled by supportive leaders (usually the Head of Midwifery) as some were employed specifically to develop, manage, and oversee this component of midwifery practice. Others used their senior position to collaborate with colleagues and senior leaders to drive the change. Either way, their roles involved ongoing collaboration and negotiation with the wider multidisciplinary teams (obstetrics, paediatrics, legal departments) and the midwives who were expected to deliver the care.

   The midwives' roles situated them in a unique position in the organisation. For example, they were a senior member of staff, yet not a manager. They had extensive clinical experience yet were not deemed as front-line workers as much of their work was 'behind the scenes'. Most of the midwives were consultant midwives, yet not part of the collective obstetric consultant teams. They were midwives, but worked across the settings (hospital, community, specialist midwives, research) and often not in a hands-on clinical way. As these midwives often worked alone, some reported feeling lonely and isolated. As such, there were multiple sources of 'us and them' (Link & Phelan, 2001) as they could be viewed as 'deviant' across the different professional groups including clinical midwives 'on the ground'. Therefore, this required proactive engagement to overcome such labelling. Their seniority and/or role, alongside the support of their leaders, may have offered some protection against the negative effects of being labelled or stereotyped:

> ... I would say that it has taken me a long time to forge those relationships with them. I've found me being clinically visible and constantly supporting women for example I am constantly in the antenatal clinic supporting women, going to meetings with the consultants, bringing cases to the consultants, talking with the cases with the consultants, it's taken a lot of leg work to get there... that's really just part and parcel of culture change, isn't it? and no it's not always been like that I think there has been inroads I suppose you know I didn't forge the way completely, there were inroads but uhm yea it has taken a lot of time and its onerous when it does end up coming down to one individual and I know the wider supervisory team does support but often we have different opinions so uh yea makes it a little bit more challenging, can be very isolating too
>
> *[Isabel]*

Whilst most of the midwives in this domain reported the occurrence of positive cultural changes across obstetric, paediatric, legal and management teams, they also reported that front-line clinical midwives delivering the care plans were a major source of resistance. Such resistance was reported to be attributed to fears of accountability, or of being blamed or scapegoated in the event of a poor outcome. Most of the midwives in this domain empathised with the front-line staff and commented all staff needed a sense of *'professional safety'* and trust in a non-punitive culture to overcome their resistance to change: '... the sense of anger amongst the community team was actually quite palpable [in relation to delivering complex homebirth care plans], and now it is something that is accepted and it's something normal' [Hannah].

These midwives worked to instil change which included the formalisation of care pathways, systems of referrals and care plans. These processes were viewed as a method of 'legitimising' women's choices and provided a physical indicator of a cultural shift occurring. Moreover, the formalisation processes were also viewed as support mechanisms for clinical staff delivering the care. Visual artefacts such as new guidelines, pathways and referral processes symbolised the new 'social contracts' put in place (Misztal, 1996), meaning the clinical staff could rely on organisational support for delivering such care:

> … I think it [care plan] empowers midwives to support women whereas maybe they, some midwives are more nervous about it, but if they have this robust plan, it empowers them …
>
> *[Jenny]*

Optimal normalised practice

This domain represented the thirteen midwives whose normal midwifery practice facilitated women's alternative choices; practices also reflected the cultural norm of their teams and across their organisations. Being a change agent was less important for those working within this domain because, in their local situation, birthing women and people's choices were already authentically embedded within the organisation. These midwives appeared to work in organisations that had reached critical mass across the professional groups and organisational structures. Some tensions or conflicts may have arisen, but these appeared to be the exception rather than the norm. The midwives seemed able to work around resistant colleagues with minimal effort:

> … so I think yes we do, we might have uhm, you could say a bit of conflict maybe if the medics are like 'why is this woman having her baby at home in the first place' sort of thing, but… usually we don't come across too many problems really …
>
> *[Anna]*

Of note, this domain was populated by midwives from a range of settings (community/hospital), with varying years' experience and levels of seniority. Therefore, the notion of 'normalised practice' was not ascribed to an individual or a team – it was characterised across the organisation. Optimal normalised practice appeared to reflect an alignment of values between the midwives' preferred woman-centred practice and their immediate and wider multi-disciplinary teams. The everyday normality of respecting women's choices was represented by effective collaborative and multi-disciplinary working, supportive and accessible care pathways, and referral or care planning processes embedded across the maternity services. Strong, supportive leadership valuing both women's choices and midwives' autonomy was present in all of the midwives' accounts – highlighted by Sam:

> Our matron and our Trust [organisation] are very pro-homebirth and is every pro woman's choice, so you kind of have her support for these women who don't fit the guidelines, you know they're not textbook women kind of thing. Her attitude is 'as long as they know the risks and you've had the conversation'…

Midwives in this domain characterised 'normalcy' (Misztal, 2001) within *'good team dynamics'* across intra and inter-professional groups marked by non-hierarchal working structures and approachable doctors and/or senior members of staff who were respectful of women's decisions and the midwives' professional autonomy. This furthered open and constructive communication and positive collaborative working across the professional groups. Mutual respect, cooperation and reciprocity appeared to be a product (Garfinkel, 1963) and an outcome (Misztal, 2001) of women's choices being 'normalised'. Kerry's account exemplified positive intra and inter-professional collaborative working:

> … when I first joined the Trust [organisation] when I had the time, I used to go these weekly meetings with the doctors, registrars and midwives who would go through the cases of women on the ward and would go through the plan and say like 'is there any other options? has anybody heard of this before?' and that really blew me away, it's not all wonderful (laughing) there are definitely a few that are and midwives that aren't perfect but there are some really good aspects of encouraging communication.

Mutually reinforced 'collective representations' [of the organisation] sustained by 'interactional rituals' (Goffman, 1963) appeared to strengthen the normalised culture. So much so, some participants referred to new members of staff *'being shocked'* to the apparent 'permissive' culture as highlighted in Chapter 5. In those situations, new members of staff were reported to be socialised quickly into adopting the organisational values with a reframed sense of 'normalcy' (Misztal, 2001). The socialisation process also included the midwives' knowledge and skill sets. For example, the midwives in this domain often cited confidence and competence in their own skill set when caring for women with complex needs. The midwives then promoted a normalised culture by providing new midwives with ongoing support and enhanced learning opportunities to gain the skills necessary to deliver such care. By not limiting new midwives' exposure to women's alternative birthing choices, the midwives created 'virtuous circles' (Downe, 2010) – furthering a woman-centred agenda.

A new perspective

This chapter has reexplored the midwives' experiences of delivering alternative physiological birth care using theoretical insights of normal/stigma, deviance/positive deviance. A spectrum from stigmatised to normalised practice illuminates the stark differences between the midwives' experiences as mediated by their micro, meso and macro working contexts. This theoretical model provides a way to account for the whole dataset to explain the findings shared in Chapters 3–5. For those experiencing the fullest expression of being perceived as 'deviant', resulted in stigmatisation with long-lasting negative repercussions. They were in an unsupportive non-negotiable working environment and faced significant challenges when enacting their preferred midwifery. Others fearful of such stigmatisation had to manage perceptions of 'deviant' behaviour and could give rise to moral distress if unable to fully support every woman's decision. For some, protective factors were identified through working in like-minded teams buffering against wider negative perceptions. Or uniquely, those viewed as advantageous to the organisation avoided negative repercussions; these midwives were labelled as 'different', however, this labelling was not detrimental. Change agents working as positive deviants had a different experience – they needed to manage the buy-in towards improving birthing women and people's access to birth choices through cultivating psychologically safe environments to manage midwife caregivers' fears and concerns. For those working in normalised cultures where women's birth choices were supported throughout the organisation, the midwives worked within a negotiable space, were supported in their practice and thus, were in optimal environments. Such environments were characterised by a positive organisational culture where delivering individualised care was viewed as a collective responsibility, not an individual (and risky) burden on one midwife. This latter point is crucial. Most childbearing women in high-income countries receive institutional care, therefore, it is essential for (holistic) safety outcomes and to deliver care women want, that care is a team effort and a collective responsibility. The next chapter focuses on institutional insights, the constraints, protective factors and enablers to present key learning messages for application at organisational levels.

Notes

1 Normal appearances relate to behavioural attributes not facial/body features, although facial/body features can also be a component.
2 Also see (Doyle & Molix, 2018; Meyer, 2003; Thoits & Link, 2015).
3 For those with visible 'stigmas', this can be a particularly difficult and a significant source of stress (Frost, 2011).
4 Also see (Swim & Thomas, 2006; Thoits & Link, 2015).
5 Also see (Wardell et al., 2018).
6 Also see (Frost & Meyer, 2012; Kumar et al., 2015).
7 Also see (Farrugia, 2009; Riggle et al., 2008; Savio, 2016).
8 Also see (Baxter et al., 2019; Heckert & Heckert, 2002; Lawton et al., 2014; Shoenberger et al., 2015).
9 Also see (Goldenberg, 2010; Rogers, 2004).

References

Adler, P. A., & Adler, P. (2015). *Constructions of Deviance: Social Power, Context, and Interaction* (8th ed.). Wadsworth.

Baxter, R., Taylor, N., Kellar, I., & Lawton, R. (2019). A qualitative positive deviance study to explore exceptionally safe care on medical wards for older people. *BMJ Quality and Safety*, 28(8), 618–626. doi: 10.1136/bmjqs-2018-008023

Berg, M. (2000). Guidelines, professionals and the production of objectivity: Standardisation and the professionalism of insurance medicine. *Sociology of Health and Illness*, 22(6), 765–791.

Beyer, M., von Scheve, C., & Sven, I. (2014). The social consequences of collective emotions 1 The Social Consequences of Collective Emotions: National Identification, Solidarity, and Out-Group Derogation. In G. Sullivan (Ed.), *Understanding Collective Pride and Group Identity: New Directions in Emotion Theory, Research and Practice* (pp. 67–80). Routledge.

Bradley, E. H., Curry, L. A., Ramanadhan, S., Rowe, L., Nembhard, I. M., & Krumholz, H. M. (2009). Research in action: Using positive deviance to improve quality of health care. *BMC Implementation Science*, 4(1). doi: 10.1186/1748-5908-4-25

Campbell, C., & Deacon, H. (2006). Unravelling the contexts of stigma: From internalisation to resistance to change. *Journal of Community and Applied Social Psychology*, 16(6), 411–417. doi: 10.1002/casp.901

Crocker, J., & Major, B. (1989). Social stigma and self-esteem: The self-protective properties of stigma. *Psychological Review*, 96(4), 608–630. doi: 10.1037/0033-295X.96.4.608

Dodge, D. L. (1985). The over Negativized conceptualization of deviance: A programmatic exploration. *Deviant Behaviour*, 6(1), 17–37. doi: 10.1080/01639625.1985.9967657

Downe, S. (2010). Beyond evidence-based medicine: Complexity and stories of maternity care. *Journal of Evaluation in Clinical Practice*, 16(1), 232–237. doi: 10.1111/j.1365-2753.2009.01357.x

Doyle, D. M., & Molix, L. (2018). Stigma consciousness modulates cortisol reactivity to social stress in women. 48(2), 217–224. doi: 10.1002/ejsp.2310

Durkheim, É. (1995). *The Elementary Forms of Religious Life*. The Free Press.

Edmondson, A. (1999). Psychological safety and learning behavior in work teams. *Administrative Science Quarterly*, 44(2), 350–383. doi: 10.2307/2666999

Farrugia, D. (2009). Exploring stigma: Medical knowledge and the stigmatisation of parents of children diagnosed with autism spectrum disorder. *Sociology of Health & Illness*, 31(7), 1011–1027. doi: 10.1111/j.1467-9566.2009.01174.x

Foucault, M. (1975). *Discipline and Punish: The Birth of the Prison*. Vintage.

Frost, D. (2011). Social Stigma and its consequences for the socially stigmatized. *Social and Personality Psychology Compass*, 5(11), 824–839. doi: 10.1111/j.1751-9004.2011.00394.x

Frost, D., & Meyer, I. (2012). Measuring community connectedness among diverse sexual minority populations. *Journal of Sex Research*, 49(1), 36–49. doi: 10.1080/00224499.2011.565427

Garfinkel, H. (1963). Motivation and social interaction cognitive determinants. In O. Harvey (Ed.), *Motivation and Social Interaction* (pp. 187–238). Ronald.

Goffman, E. (1963). *Stigma. Notes on the Management of Spoiled Identity*. Prentice Hall.

Goffman, E. (1971). *Relations in Public: Microstudies of the Public Order*. Basic Books.

Goldenberg, M. (2010). Perspectives on evidence-based healthcare for women. *Journal of Women's Health*, 19(7), 1235–1238. doi: 10.1089/jwh.2009.1680

Hayward, L. E., Vartanian, L. R., & Pinkus, R. T. (2018). Weight stigma predicts poorer psychological well-being through internalized weight bias and maladaptive coping responses. *Obesity: A Research Journal*, 26(4), 755–761. doi: 10.1002/oby.22126

Heckert, A., & Heckert, D. M. (2002). A new typology of deviance: Integrating normative and reactivist definitions of deviance. *Deviant Behavior*, 23(5), 449–479. doi: 10.1080/016396202320265319

Herek, G. M. (2009). Hate crimes and stigma-related experiences among sexual minority adults in the United States: Prevalence estimates from a national probability sample. *Journal of Interpersonal Violence*, 24(1), 54–74. doi: 10.1177/0886260508316477

Herington, M. J., & van de Fliert, E. (2018). Positive deviance in theory and practice: A conceptual review. *Deviant Behavior*. 39(5), 664–678. doi: 10.1080/01639625.2017.1286194

Kumar, S., Mohanraj, R., Rao, D., Murray, K. R., & Manhart, L. E. (2015). Positive coping strategies and HIV-related stigma in South India. *AIDS Patient Care and STDs*, 29(3), 157–163. doi: 10.1089/apc.2014.0182

Lawton, R., Taylor, N., Clay-Williams, R., & Braithwaite, J. (2014). Positive deviance: A different approach to achieving patient safety. *BMJ Quality & Safety*, 23(11), 880–883. doi: 10.1136/bmjqs-2014-003115

Link, B. G., & Phelan, J. C. (2001). Conceptualizing stigma. *Annual Review of Sociology*, 27(1), 363–385. doi: 10.1146/annurev.soc.27.1.363

Luhmann, N. (2000). Familiarity, confidence, trust: Problems and alternatives. In D. Gambetta (Ed.), *Trust: Making and Breaking Cooperative Relations* (pp. 94–107). University of Oxford.

Meyer, I. H. (2003). Prejudice as stress: Conceptual and measurement problems. *American Journal of Public Health*, 93(2), 262–265. doi: 10.2105/AJPH.93.2.262

Misztal, B. (1996). *Trust in Modern Societies: The Search for the Bases of Social Order* (1st ed.). Polity Press.

Misztal, B. (2001). Normality and trust in Goffman's theory of interaction order. *Sociological Theory*, 19(3), 312–324.

Ortashi, O., Virdee, J., Hassan, R., Mutrynowski, T., & Abu-Zidan, F. (2013). The practice of defensive medicine among hospital doctors in the United Kingdom. *BMC Medical Ethics*, 14(1). doi: 10.1186/1472-6939-14-42

Phelan, J., Link, B., & Dovidio, J. (2008). Stigma and prejudice: One animal or two? *Social Science & Medicine*, 67(3), 358–367. doi: 10.1016/j.socscimed.2008.03.022

Riggle, E. D. B., Whitman, J. S., Olson, A., Rostosky, S. S., & Strong, S. (2008). The positive aspects of being a lesbian or gay man. 39(2), 210–217. doi: 10.1037/0735-7028.39.2.210

Rock, L. (2007). The good mother vs. the other mother: The girl-mom. *Journal of the Motherhood Initiative for Research and Community Involvement*, 9(1), 20–28.

Rogers, W. (2004). Evidence-based medicine and women: Do the principles and practice of EBM further women's health? *Bioethics*, 18(1), 50–71. doi: 10.1111/j.1467-8519.2004.00378.x

Sabel, C. F. (1993). Studied trust: Building new forms of cooperation in a volatile economy. *Human Relations*, 46(9), 1133–1170. doi: 10.1177/001872679304600907

Savio, G. (2016). Organization and stigma management: A comparative study of dumpster divers in New York. *Sociological Perspectives*, 60(2), 416–430. doi: 10.1177/0731121416632012

Scott, J. (1999). Geographies of trust, geographies of hierarchies. In M. Warrent (Ed.), *Democracy and Trust* (pp. 273–289). Cambridge University Press.

Sheppard, B. H., & Sherman, D. M. (1998). The grammars of trust: A model and general implications. *Academy of Management Review*, 23(3), 422–437. doi: 10.2307/259287

Shih, M. (2004). Positive stigma: Examining resilience and empowerment in overcoming stigma. *The ANNALS of the American Academy of Political and Social Science*, 591(1), 175–202.

Shoenberger, N., Heckert, A., & Heckert, D. (2015). Labeling, social learning, and positive deviance: A look at high achieving students. *Deviant Behavior*, 36(6), 474–491. doi: 0.1080/01639625.2014.944066

Singhal, A., & Dura, L. (2017). Positive deviance: A non-normative approach to health and risk messaging. *Oxford Research Encyclopedias*. doi: 10.1093/acrefore/9780190228613.013.248

Spreitzer, G., & Sonenshein, S. (2003). Positive deviance and extraordinary organizing. In K. Cameron, J. Dutton & R. Quinn (Eds.), *Positive Organisational Scholarship* (pp. 207–224). Berrett-Koehler.

Swim, J. K., & Thomas, M. A. (2006). Responding to everyday discrimination: A synthesis of research on goal-directed, self-regulatory coping behaviors. In S. Levin & C. van Laar (Eds.), *Stigma and Group Inequality: Social Psychological Perspectives* (pp. 105–126). Lawrence Erlbaum Associates Publishers.

Thoits, P. (1995). Stress, coping, and social support processes: Where are we? What next? *Journal of Health and Social Behavior*, 53–79. https://www.jstor.org/stable/2626957?origin=crossref

Thoits, P., & Link, B. (2015). Stigma resistance and well-being among people in treatment for psychosis. *Society and Mental Health*, 6(1), 1–20. doi: 10.1177/2156869315591367

Unger, R. (1998). Positive marginality: Antecedents and consequences. *Journal of Adult Development*, 5(3), 163–170.

Wardell, J. D., Shuper, P. A., Rourke, S. B., & Hendershot, C. S. (2018). Stigma, coping, and alcohol use severity among people living with HIV: A prospective analysis of bidirectional and mediated associations. *Annals of Behavioral Medicine*, 52(9), 762–772. doi: 10.1093/abm/kax050

7

SHIFTING THE LENS

Towards a collective responsibility

The previous chapter presented a theoretical model 'stigmatised – normalised' practice, a reinterpretation of the data using theories of stigma/normal, deviance/positive deviance. These theories accounted for the whole dataset to explore and explain the sociocultural-political workplace influences on the midwives' practice when supporting alternative physiological births. Where Chapter 3 demonstrated how midwives facilitated these births, Chapters 4–6 illuminated the polarised spectrum of experiences of doing so, as mediated by their working contexts. Crucially, those working in supportive environments were not individually burdened by challenging sociocultural-political contexts to practice woman-centred care. Rather, their organisational culture was characterised by collective responsibility to meet the needs of birthing women and people. As such, the midwives were enabled to practice autonomously within a psychologically safe culture. This chapter explores the key messages from the study, drawing on the wider literature to provide a framework to understand the constraints, protective factors and enablers of supporting alternative physiological birthing choices (see Figure 7.1). Critically, the enabling factors cited in the latter part of the chapter demonstrate the positive relationship between enabling workplace environments and birthing women and people receiving supportive maternity care. Organisations led by compassionate, collective leadership upholding values of maternal autonomy and trust within their staff perpetuate virtuous cycles benefiting staff and service users alike. Not least because staff wellbeing is directly correlated with improved outcomes, but also because supportive, psychologically safe environments protect workforce sustainability. Given the dire staffing situation, these insights are crucial when considering recruitment and retention.

DOI: 10.4324/9781003265443-7

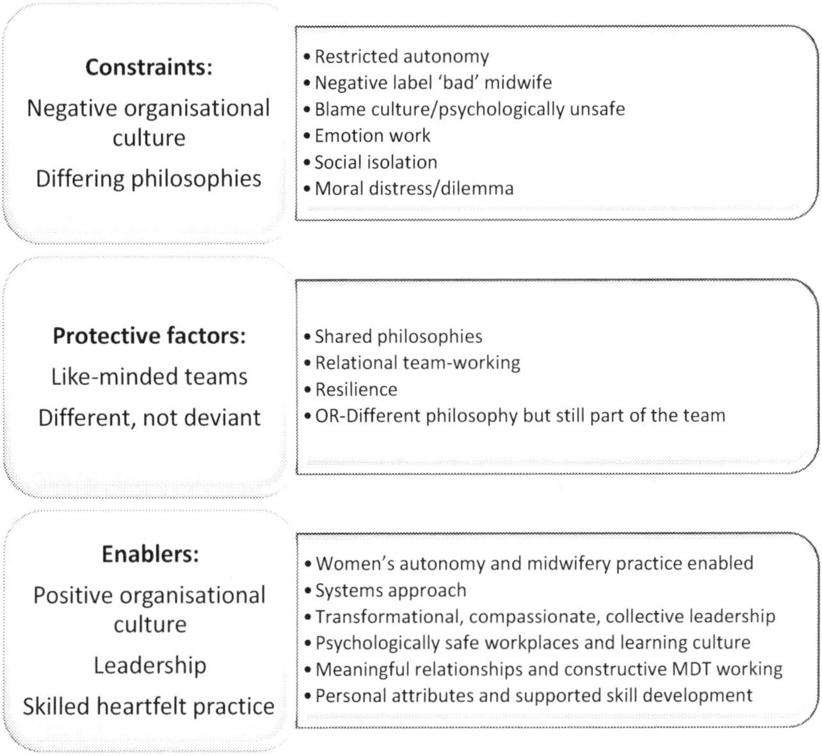

Constraints:

Negative organisational culture

Differing philosophies

- Restricted autonomy
- Negative label 'bad' midwife
- Blame culture/psychologically unsafe
- Emotion work
- Social isolation
- Moral distress/dilemma

Protective factors:

Like-minded teams

Different, not deviant

- Shared philosophies
- Relational team-working
- Resilience
- OR-Different philosophy but still part of the team

Enablers:

Positive organisational culture

Leadership

Skilled heartfelt practice

- Women's autonomy and midwifery practice enabled
- Systems approach
- Transformational, compassionate, collective leadership
- Psychologically safe workplaces and learning culture
- Meaningful relationships and constructive MDT working
- Personal attributes and supported skill development

FIGURE 7.1 Constraints, protective factors, and enablers.

Constraints

Understanding the organisational constraints midwives faced when supporting alternative physiological births adds to the body of evidence around why midwives leave, and the barriers women and birthing people face when asserting their agency. This study has provided nuanced insights when the essence of midwifery philosophy and practice are perceived as threatening at an organisational level. Moreover, these findings have demonstrated the barriers midwives face regarding autonomy, belonging and contribution as per the King's Fund (2020) ABC model. With patient experiences of care and outcomes strongly associated with staff wellbeing (Nembhard & Edmondson, 2006; West et al., 2014), it can be deduced for those seeking alternative physiological births where midwives are *not* supported, their access to, and experiences of care are likely poorer.

Negative organisational culture

The issues raised in Chapters 4 and 6 specifically related to organisational *culture* as problematic, rather than those typically found in other studies such as staffing, resources, workload or busyness (Ball et al., 2003; RCM, 2016; RCM, 2018). Organisational culture defined by Davies et al. (2000) as 'a pattern of shared beliefs and values that gives members of an institution meaning and provides them with the rules for behaviour in their organisation' (p. 112) can also be identified as 'the way things are done around here', how things are understood, judged or valued. For some of the midwives in this study, negative organisational cultures were distinguished by a patriarchal culture permeating all levels of the organisation. Characterised by poor leadership, lack of embedded (tacit or documented) pathways to support women's choices, unsupportive management and/or obstetric staff, and a lack of peer support. These cultures prioritised the operational processes within medicalised and guideline-centric discourses, over evidence-based medicine, client and midwifery autonomy. Thus, mirroring the broader criticisms explored in Chapter 2 (over-medicalisation and guideline-centred care). An over-medicalised and 'guideline-centred' (Kotaska, 2011) approach to care contradicts the values of evidence-based medicine (Wieringa, 2017), the legal standing of women's autonomy (Birthrights, 2013), midwifery philosophy of individualised care (ICM, 2014), national maternity guidelines (NICE, 2017), government maternity policies (NHS England, 2016) and international agendas of respectful maternity care (White Ribbon Alliance, 2011). Such contradictions appeared prevalent in some cases, despite the known limitations of guidelines (Gabbay, 2004) and the iatrogenic harms caused by an over-medicalised approach to birth (Miller et al., 2016).

Restrictive autonomy reduced the midwives' ability to practice 'full-scope' midwifery (Renfrew et al., 2014) and is likely to reduce women's access to birth choices. Beyond obvious restrictions such as discriminatory or punitive actions (seen in Chapters 4 and 6), restrictive autonomy could occur more subtly. For example, situations where the midwife faced numerous obstacles or 'hoops' to jump through and where access to supportive teams was withheld (see Chapter 4). Moreover, patriarchal organisational cultures were reinforced through deviant labelling (Dodge, 1985) – 'a bad or dangerous midwife'. A bad midwife was implicitly or explicitly viewed as one who actively encouraged women to make 'dangerous choices'. As a detrimental stigmatising label (Goffman, 1963) bad midwifery mirrors the patriarchal binary 'good/bad' mother discourses (Goodwin & Huppatz, 2010). These discourses situate 'good mothers' as women who with 'docile bodies, will not resist or question the 'experts'' (Rock, 2007, p. 21). Applied to the midwives, a 'good midwife' could be perceived as the efficient (docile) worker that values the institutional needs over women's, one that does not resist or question organisational structures. Thus, the midwives were 'othered' which served to discredit the midwife and fostered feelings of fear and vulnerability – a method of control reinforcing hierarchies (Foucault, 1975). Therefore, organisational cultures which stigmatise midwives who work within an authentically woman-centred philosophy can catalyse severe adverse consequences for those midwives. This is a significant barrier for those midwives to deliver the kind of care embedded in their professional rules and codes of practice.

Issues of negative organisational cultures also related to notions of a 'blame' culture (Robertson & Thomson, 2016), where punitive rather than restorative action was the norm. A 'blame' culture is characterised by investigations that focus upon individual fault, rather than system failures (Woodward, 2022) and seek to determine personal negligence in response to potential litigation (Robertson & Thomson, 2016). A blame culture is suggested to reduce practitioner's openness and transparency in the event of mistakes and is cited as causing fear in practitioners with detrimental impacts on their emotional well-being (Alexander & Bogossian, 2018), causing a loss of confidence (Robertson & Thomson, 2016; Wier, 2017) and can increase defensive clinical practice (Ortashi et al., 2013; Wier, 2017). As found in this study, fears of undue accountability, negligence, and litigation coalesced to create restrictions for women and midwives facilitating alternative birthing choices. For those who resisted negative organisational culture, and, as a result, risked or experienced persistent stigmatisation and reprisals for their practice (even where poor outcomes did not occur). Despite these challenges most of the midwives affected continued to exercise their sense of moral vocation; their values and alignment with supporting women's access to skilled midwifery care served as a resistance to the dominant culture of fear and blame.

Disparities of philosophies

Disparities between the midwives' philosophy of care and their colleagues created significant tensions, constrained the midwives' practice and created 'emotion work' (Hunter, 2004) – the work involved in managing emotions in the workplace (Hoschschild, 1983). A strong misalignment between the midwives' practice and their colleagues, caused excessive 'emotion work' and was a significant source of distress (Chapter 4). Moreover, the disparities between midwifery philosophies risked the study participants being labelled and/or stereotyped as 'deviant' resulting in social isolation, vulnerability and stress (Hunter, 2010; Kirkham et al., 2002; RCM, 2016). Such bullying in the workplace mirrors the wider literature around horizontal violence in midwifery (Leap, 1997) and reinforces hierarchical institutional norms (Foucault, 1975). In this study, social isolation, a form of bullying, was specifically related to clashes between midwifery values, contextualised by organisational cultures unsupportive of women's and/or midwives' autonomy. Moreover, fears of being labelled and stigmatised also created stress through 'stigma management' (Goffman, 1963) (see Chapter 6), hence, managing these tensions was another source of emotion work for the midwives (Hunter, 2010). Strained collegial relationships have been identified in other studies as a source of distress and challenge (Deery & Kirkham, 2007; Hunter, 2005). Moreover, this study demonstrated the subsequent ill effects of poor working relationships and/or bullying as found in other studies; stress, burnout, health problems, mental-emotional distress, taking time off sick, leaving jobs and leaving the profession (Hunter, 2005).[1] Such psychologically unsafe environments are in direct contrast to the King's Fund (2020) recommendations of what midwives need to flourish.

The misalignment between the midwives', their colleagues and/or organisational philosophies contributed to 'battles' to deliver woman-centred care, mirroring the wider literature which has found midwives suffer when they are unable to deliver appropriate good care (Hunter & Warren, 2014).[2] The midwives displayed simultaneous challenge to and reinforcement of the status quo. Akin to the ethnographic findings by Pollard (2011) who investigated midwives' discursive practices in a labour ward and found they revealed inconsistent identities – sometimes challenging medicalised and professional hierarchies but at other times, reinforcing the status quo. However, the midwives in this study highlighted their rationale for managing their identities and practice to cope with interprofessional tensions through sacrificing some of their values they were able to (mostly) retain collegial working relationships and often meet the needs of women in their care (though not always). Juggling ethical dilemmas of which battle to fight and adopting a discerning approach, provided some protection to continue to practice their preferred midwifery most of the time. However, the ongoing ethical dilemmas of which battle to fight created 'moral distress' – knowing the ethically correct thing to do but feeling unable to act (Jameton, 1984). In this light, significant concerns are raised regarding the long-term impact of managing persistent ethical sacrifices and moral dilemmas – a factor why midwives leave the profession. Moreover, it raises ethical issues and dilemmas for the midwives of who to offer 'extras' to, as the midwife is unlikely to be able to offer the same level of care to all women. Thus, potentially leading to inequitable care provision and divisions between women.

Protective factors

Within the context of workplace constraints, some midwives had protection against the negative effects of poor and unsupportive work environments. This contributes to understanding why or how midwives may stay – as employees of a specific institution and more broadly, staying within the profession. The valuable protective roles of being in 'supportive like-minded teams' and where midwives were perceived as 'different but not deviant' within their workplaces were protective factors. Both connect to the King's Fund (2020) ABC framework for what midwives need. Despite broader challenging workplace cultures, these protective factors created some space for autonomy, belonging and contribution (King's Fund, 2020). Moreover, some psychological safety was present for these midwives. For those working in like-minded teams, their intra-team relationships provided enough shelter from broader workplace challenges, and a safe space to share challenges and garner support. For those midwives simply accepted by their team members as 'one of those midwives' psychological safety was generated by this acceptance of their midwifery practice, not viewed as a threat, but as a benefit to their teammates. Therefore, these midwives were able to work within their values without fear of repercussion.

Supportive like-minded teams

A key protective factor and source of resilience were working in like-minded and supportive teams. Feeling supported and understood created a shared identity and a sense of belonging – protecting the midwives from the ill effects of negative labelling or stereotyping (Link & Phelan, 2001). Working with those with a similar ethos, midwives were enabled and empowered to practice woman-centred care. Whilst negative situations did occur, the teams dealt with them together, thus sharing the 'burden'. Consequently, my study identified that the midwives' source of social capital[3] was generated by 'horizontal trust (employee to employee) and reciprocity' Hunter (2010). This mostly fulfilled their needs for autonomy, belonging and contribution (King's Fund, 2020) as strong relationships between team members, working as a cohesive unit mitigated against the broader institutional constraints. The benefits of strong team relationships have been found in other studies and within international contexts – the UK, Australia and New Zealand. Collectively, they demonstrated why midwives stay in the profession and provide insights into sustainable midwifery practice. For example, 'family-like' relationships are characterised by mutual support and friendships (Walsh, 2007), positive collegial interactions and a sense of belonging (Sullivan et al., 2011). Working with supportive teams (Catling et al., 2017) and working with like-minded colleagues (Crowther et al., 2016) all have been found to contribute to positive working environments and are mitigating factors against difficult workplace cultures. As sources of resilience, positive relational team working is an essential component to facilitate the midwives' ability to practice 'full-scope' midwifery, and crucially, for women and birthing people to get their needs met.

Different, not deviant

Conversely, protective factors also existed for individual midwives who were practising authentic woman-centred care but where it was not the cultural norm. As an anomaly across the dataset, these midwives were perceived as 'different' rather than 'deviant'. Not seen as threatening, was a strong protective factor against negative labelling or stereotyping. Moreover, they felt it to be beneficial to their team or organisation. Situated as a midwife suited to a 'type of woman', these midwives lessened the workload for their colleagues who preferred not to care for women making alternative birthing choices. Therefore, the midwives had a valued position within their working social groups. Being accepted by their teams, despite their different midwifery philosophy, could be explained by the midwives' extensive clinical experience and long-time standing within their organisations. They were trusted and respected – largely left to 'get on with it'. Having built working relationships with their colleagues over extended periods suggests 'being known', protected the midwives from negative stereotyping. Therefore, they cultivated positive working relationships, offering a unique insight into the nature of midwifery practice where philosophies amongst colleagues differ, demonstrating it may not always be disadvantageous.

Enablers

Offering a positive counter-discourse, other midwives in this study experienced positive workplaces not conforming to the issues highlighted in Chapter 2. Crucially, these midwives worked across the settings including the community, birth centres and hospitals. Thus, reflecting wider positive organisational cultures supportive of both women's choices and midwives to deliver the care, and were not limited to particular silos or settings. Understanding these enabling factors offers insights for midwifery workforce retention. Within the ABC framework (King's Fund, 2020) these findings show how a structural, systems approach to supporting women's choices shifts the lens from an individual 'burden' of fulfilling women's choices to that of a collective (system-wide) responsibility. In this way, the midwives had their autonomy enabled, belonged to a wider supportive culture, and found ways to express their contributions through their work of supporting alternative physiological birth choices. The systemic approach was characterised by mutual respect, trust, and open communication across the organisation. For those within change agent roles, their job was to create enabling environments to help shift the culture – using compassionate, transformational leadership approaches to facilitate organisational-wide, cultural change. These enabling factors, highlight the core principles of an 'enabling environment' as defined by the International Confederation of Midwives (2021) as *'an environment which values and respects midwives and values and respects women p.6'.* This definition means the workplace environment facilitates midwives to practice to their full scope, midwives have access to continuing professional development and career pathways, work within a functional health infrastructure, have access to timely and respectful consultation and collaboration, are safe from physical and emotional harm and have fair equitable compensation and working conditions (ICM, 2021). All of which are highlighted below.

Positive organisational culture

Woman and person-centred organisational values and culture created the optimal environment for midwives to deliver woman-centred care where women's (alternative) choices were 'normalised'. Central to this was a lack of tension between birthing women and people's autonomy and the needs of the organisations. Moreover, midwives were trusted to deliver this type of care and retain high levels of autonomy (Doherty & O'Brien, 2022). Midwives reported ongoing and accessible support when caring for women making alternative choices across the continuum; antenatal care planning, intrapartum and/or postnatal care. Additionally, colleague debriefing was valued and appeared to facilitate the delivery of woman-centred care. Where midwives had access to supportive, non-judgemental peers or senior staff they reported greater confidence in delivering woman-centred care. In keeping with definitions of 'organisational cultures' outlined earlier (Davies et al., 2000), positive organisational cultures were characterised by: valuing women's autonomy, strong and supportive leadership, positive and trusting intra and inter-professional relationships, and embedded, accessible pathways or processes utilised across the organisation. Collectively, the positive organisational cultures enhanced multi-disciplinary team working e.g., fostering constructive positive inter-professional relationships is a hallmark of safe maternity services (Liberati et al., 2019) and positive working cultures (Doherty & O'Brien, 2022) and reduces the likelihood of workplace burnout which, in turn, reduces staff turnover and absenteeism (Hunter et al., 2019; Smith, 2021). All of this is likely to have a positive impact on care experienced by women and birthing people. Therefore, learning from those working within positive organisational cultures is vital to understanding well-functioning maternity units so others can improve.

Moreover, in contrast to a 'blame' culture, these midwives worked within 'learning cultures' (Crowe & Manley, 2019). Where blame cultures have been observed as creating toxic cultures, the opposite is true in authentic learning cultures as found in this study. Openness, honesty and transparency are all characteristics of psychologically safe, learning workplace environments (Crowe & Manley, 2019; Edmondson, 1999). Therefore, when mistakes are made (not if, but when, as all high-stakes environments will encounter human errors), staff can be honest without fear of punitive repercussions (West et al., 2017) enhancing the safety of organisations, as mistakes caught early can be rectified and lessons learnt rapidly (Liberati et al., 2019). Trust was central to the learning cultures found in this study whereby delivering a safe service required a cohesive (trusting) team and psychological safety was explicit. These positive attributes, enhanced their teamwork communication and effectiveness while maintaining workforce sustainability (lack of psychological safety increases stressors, the likelihood of burnout and attrition) (Edmondson, A. & Harvey, 2017; Nembhard & Edmondson, 2006; O'Donovan & McAuliffe, 2020a). In terms of alternative physiological births, which may create greater vulnerability for some maternity staff, within an open learning no-blame culture such as the environments highlighted in this study, staff could be supported to work outside of their comfort zones to meaningfully support an array of birth choices. In this way, women, birthing people, midwives and all maternity staff have their autonomy enabled through a system-wide approach.

Transformational, compassionate, collective leadership

For respondents who were situated as change agents, being in or securing a leadership role facilitated improvements to the services. Organisational change was facilitated by working in collaboration with the multi-disciplinary team and midwifery caregivers demonstrated through transformation, compassionate and collective leadership approaches (Chapter 5). However, the change agents had to provide meaningful structures, tacit and practical, to overcome resistance from midwife caregivers to address their fears and concerns (Feeley et al., 2019). Where caregivers were particularly resistant, visual artefacts such as care pathways endorsed by the organisation combined with direct support from the change agents facilitated positive cultural changes. These approaches and visual artefacts helped 'prove' institutional support was authentic and available, enhancing psychologically safe cultures (O'Donovan & McAuliffe, 2020b). Moreover, the change makers sought to create a system-wide change to improve the overall organisational culture as this approach is vital to the improvement of just, learning cultures and better services (West et al., 2014). A scoping review carried out by Frith et al. (2014) identified several studies that sought to improve a midwifery model of maternity practice within organisational cultures with various service changes. However, none of the included studies related to changes stimulated by midwives specifically in leadership roles (specialist, supervisory or consultant midwife) as was found in this study. My study suggested midwives in senior leadership positions who were philosophically orientated toward authentic relational care were able to change organisational cultures in this direction. This was further supported by those participants who worked within positive organisational cultures, they consistently raised the importance of effective, supportive leadership to create enabling environments. Therefore, in this study we see it from both angles, driving change and where change had already occurred, how woman-centred, positive learning cultures were developed and retained. While some of the participants were consultant midwives, a role unique to the UK and Australia (Fernandez et al., 2017; Robinson, 2012), their principles of engaging with change can be applied elsewhere.

Crucial to effective cultural change were the conditions in which leaders created an 'emotionally and professionally safe' environment for the midwife caregivers including access to support and help, a learning (not blame) culture and a visible demonstration of leadership. Having discussed psychological safety at great length (see Chapter 5), we can expand on this to consider it as a relational approach to leadership to cultivating psychological safety in the workplace. Such a relational approach to leadership can be viewed within transformational leadership theory – one model by Kouzes & Posner (2011) suggests there are five domains of transformational leadership; 1. 'Model the way' relates to leaders developing their own values and setting an example for others. 2. 'Inspire a shared vision' relates to leaders developing an exciting vision which inspires others. 3. 'Challenge the process' relating to innovations, experiments and risk-taking. 4. 'Enable others to act' relates to fostering collaborations and empowering others to act. 5. 'Encourage the heart' relates to recognition and acknowledgement of others' achievements. Viewed within a transformational leadership model, compassionate and collective leadership approaches were also present within the findings, adding qualitative insights regarding the positive benefits of consultant midwives and other specialist roles in the facilitation of change (and sustaining it) towards greater woman-centred services.

Skilled heartfelt practice

Skilled heartfelt practice denotes the interrelationship between the midwives' attitudes and ethical beliefs in support of women's choices, their values of cultivating meaningful relationships along with their practical clinical skills. Arguably, it is these qualities combined which give rise to the practice of 'full-scope midwifery' (Renfrew et al., 2014), and are an essential enabling factor to support women's alternative choices. While the nature of the workplace culture and environments were found to be enabling or hindering, the midwives' personal attributes, values and clinical skill sets were essential to delivering this care. Chapter 3 illuminated just how the midwives facilitated women's alternative physiological birthing choices – deploying a range of emotional intelligence and clinical skill sets. Moreover, midwives in this study demonstrated high levels of experience, skill, competence and confidence in their physiological birth skills which they were able to apply to out of guideline birth choices (Hunter et al., 2018). This was partly explained by their personal motivations or philosophy, actively seeking to develop their skills and competence, as well as extensive exposure to non-obstetric environments. Repeated exposure within supportive environments has been found as a key facilitator for midwives to develop confidence and competence in their skill sets (Hunter et al., 2018; Nicholls & Webb, 2006).[4] The midwives' demonstrable skills in physiological labour were also explained by the availability and accessibility of continuing professional development, refresher days, and supportive structures in which an ongoing learning environment continued to enhance the midwives' skill sets. Such environments combined with self-motivation enabled many midwives to move from 'novice to expert' practitioners (Benner, 1984). Expertise relates to the shift from the reliance upon rules and analytical thinking (novice) to inform decision-making, towards greater independence where knowledge, experience, and intuition are synthesised quickly to guide actions or decision-making (expert) (Benner, 1984).

Additionally, some situations did require specialist input or advanced knowledge e.g., caring for women with multiple morbidities, significant illnesses such as blood-borne viruses, epilepsy or insulin-controlled diabetes. In these situations, the midwives applied their midwifery knowledge of healthy women in labour to those with complicated pregnancies and sought collaboration with obstetric or specialist doctors to develop appropriate care plans. Again, repeated exposure to women with complicated pregnancies appeared to broaden their experience and enhanced their skill-sets (Nicholls & Webb, 2006; Jordan & Farley, 2008). Therefore, a systems approach must be operationalised to ensure midwives have the appropriate skills and access to continuing professional development so women receive appropriately safe and skilled care aligned with the human rights framework (ICM, 2021). Many of the midwives in this study illuminated just how this can be achieved within institutional settings.

Enabling work environments, enabling birth choices

Maternity services are tasked with providing safe, high-quality maternity care that is accessible, equitable, and critically, based on the needs of birthing women and people. Those needs span across a spectrum of choice and decision-making; from opting out of maternity care (freebirthing) to elective caesareans and everything in between. The focus of this book, this research, was to highlight the issues surrounding alternative physiological birth choices. As highlighted in Chapters 1 and 2, these birth choices can be viewed as contentious with complex sociocultural-political discourses influencing maternity service provision, maternity professionals' practice and women's access to care (or not) for these decisions. The interplay of these discourses is not unique to maternity services, for societal shifts and changes continually influence health and expectations. What is particular about maternity services is as a female-dominated professional and service user space, broader societal issues (misogyny, patriarchy, under-valuing of women's work, etc.) are distilled into the heightened time of childbearing.

That the fetus has become the 'second patient' (Doyal, 1979) we must be constantly alert to the saviour complex seeking to rescue babies from their 'dangerous' mothers (Rock, 2007). This insidious cultural shift continually attempts to erode women and childbearing people's rights and pits the mother against her child through reinforcing sex and gender-based conventions and/or constraints. Explicit or implicit messaging criticises women with the charge of seeking a birth experience over that of the safety of her child.[5] However, as Downe (cited in Dagustun) (2021)[6] reminds us, it is not either/or, it is both/and. This means we can (and should) value and serve the mother-baby dyad in its entirety, attending to both the experience and outcomes of birth. Broadly, this is what my study has shown. How midwives can and do facilitate autonomous birth decisions within a human rights framework, respecting the mother-baby dyad in terms of experience *and* outcomes demonstrated woman and person-centred care in action. The facilitation of these births was underpinned by evidence-informed care, careful planning and competence to facilitate physiological births. Central to which was relational care. Safe care *is* relational care as highlighted in this study.

However, throughout this book, the study findings have shown the significance of the midwives' workplaces – either an enabling or hindering environment. While this may appear obvious (it is), unique to this study is unpacking what this means exactly, how it plays out in everyday practice, what it looks like, feels like and of course the emotional, mental and physical impact on the midwives' wellbeing. Moreover, this study captured the views and experiences from midwives working in extremely different environments. It has included devastating accounts from midwives stigmatised for their practice, but also included inspiring accounts from midwives fully supported in their role. It is vital for the midwives working within challenging environments to feel heard and seen, and I hope this book has offered that to them, to those currently working in these types of workplaces. It is also vital we take the positive lessons of what works and how it works forward. This book offers insights others can learn from, adopt and take into their practice – an enabling workplace environments for midwives is an enabling environment for birthing women and people where their decisions are respected and upheld.

While this book focused on alternative physiological birth choices as they are the direct domain of midwives, these lessons can be applied to supporting all and any birth choices – listening, understanding, supporting, and actioning what women want is central to all ethical maternity care. However, the focus on physiological birth is an important conversation and foci. As physiological birth rates continue to fall, and if maternity services do not address the inequitable access to skilled, competent midwives to facilitate these births that women want and expect, we know from the wider research, women will stop engaging with care providers (Greenfield et al., 2021; Holten & de Miranda, 2016; McKenzie & Montgomery, 2021). Equitable access includes 24/7 homebirth and birth centre facilities fully staffed with competent, skilled practitioners, and when transfers occur[7] the MDT are supportive. It also includes competent maternity professionals understanding and working with the anatomy, physiology and psychology of birth. It means listening and meaningfully supporting women's choices, trusting midwives' autonomy, and creating psychologically safe environments where honesty, transparency and support are tangible. These conditions do not need to be at loggerheads with other maternity provisions women want, such as access to epidurals or caesarean sections. However, they do need to be valued in the same way with the same level of attention, resourcing and support. That way, we create a truly equitable maternity service, an enabling environment, meeting the needs of all women and birthing people and their midwife caregivers (ICM, 2021).

Notes

1 Also see (Ball et al., 2003; Curtis et al., 2006; Gillen et al., 2008; Hunter & Warren, 2013, 2014; Hunter et al., 2018).
2 Also see these references cited above.
3 The networks of relationships among people who live and work in a particular society, enabling that society to function effectively.
4 Also see (Jordan & Farley, 2008; Lewis & Hauck, 2018; Thompson et al., 2016).
5 UK media reporting makes explicit references to 'obsessions' or the 'cult' of natural birth – for examples, see (Daily Mail Online, 2011; Glaser, 2015).
6 Professor Soo Downe has emphasised a 'both/and' approach throughout many presentations and talks, many are available online.
7 A good opportunity to reiterate transfers from home or birth centres are a sign the system is working effectively and is safe practice (Reitsma et al., 2020) and not a sign of failure.

References

Alexander, C. R., & Bogossian, F. (2018). Midwives and clinical investigation: A review of the literature. *Women and Birth*, (6), 442–452. doi: 10.1016/j.wombi.2018.02.003

Ball, L., Curtis, P., & Kirkham, M. (2003). *Why Do Midwives Leave? Talking to the Managers.* (No. 1). London: Royal College of Midwives.

Benner, P. (1984). *From Novice to Expert: Excellence and Power in Clinical Nursing Practice.* Addison-Wesley, Menlo Park.

Birthrights. (2013). The dignity survey 2013: Women's and midwives' experiences of UK maternity care. London: Birthrights. http://www.birthrights.org.uk/wordpress/wp-content/uploads/2013/10/Birthrights-Dignity-Survey.pdf

Catling, C. J., Reid, F., & Hunter, B. (2017). Australian midwives' experiences of their workplace culture. *Women and Birth*, 30(2), 137–145. 10.1016/j.wombi.2016.10.001

Crowe, C., & Manley, K. (2019). Person-centred, safe and effective care in maternity services: The need for greater change towards best practice. *International Practice Development Journal*, 9(1), 1–20.

Crowther, S., Hunter, B., McAra-Couper, J., Warren, L., Gilkison, A., Hunter, M., Fielder, A., & Kirkham, M. (2016). Sustainability and resilience in midwifery: A discussion paper. *Midwifery*, 40, 40–48. 10.1016/j.midw.2016.06.005

Curtis, P., Ball, L., & Kirkham, M. (2006). Why do midwives leave? (not) being the kind of midwife you want to be. *British Journal of Midwifery*, 14(1), 27–31.

Dagustun, J. (2021). An interview with Soo Downe by the AIMS campaigns team. *AIMS Journal*, 33(1), 32–35.

Daily Mail Online. (2011). *Is an obsession with natural birth putting mothers and babies at risk?* Daily Mail. https://www.dailymail.co.uk/health/article-2044875/Is-obsession-natural-birth-putting-mothers-babies-danger.html

Davies, H. T., Nutley, S. M., & Mannion, R. (2000). Organisational culture and quality of health care. *BMJ Quality & Safety*, 9(2), 111–119. 10.1136/qhc.9.2.111

Deery, R., & Kirkham, M. (2007). Drained and dumped on the generation and accumulation of emotional toxic waste in community midwifery. In M. Kirkham (Ed.) *Exploring the Dirty Side of Women's Health* (pp. 72–85). Routledge.

Dodge, D. L. (1985). The over negativized conceptualization of deviance: A programmatic exploration. *Deviant Behaviour*, 6(1), 17–37. doi: 10.1080/01639625.1985.9967657

Doherty, J., & O'Brien, D. (2022). Reducing midwife burnout at organisational level — Midwives need time, space and a positive work-place culture. *Women and Birth*, In Press. doi: 10.1016/j.wombi.2022.02.003

Doyal, L. (1979). *The Political Economy of Health.* Pluto Press.

Edmondson, A. (1999). Psychological safety and learning behavior in work teams. *Administrative Science Quarterly*, 44(2), 350–383. doi: 10.2307/2666999

Edmondson, A., & Harvey, J. (2017). *Extreme Teaming: Lessons in Complex, Cross-Sector Leadership.* Emerald Group Publishing Limited.

Feeley, C., Thomson, G., & Downe, S. (2019). Caring for women making unconventional birth choices: A meta-ethnography exploring the views, attitudes, and experiences of midwives. *Midwifery*, 72, 50–59. doi: 10.1016/j.midw.2019.02.009

Fernandez, R. S., Sheppard-Law, S., & Manning, V. (2017). Determining the key drivers and mitigating factors that influence the role of the Nurse and/or Midwife Consultant: A cross-sectional survey. *Contemporary Nurse*, 53(3), 302–312. doi: 10.1080/10376178.2017.1338525

Foucault, M. (1975). *Discipline and Punish: The Birth of the Prison.* Vintage.

Frith, L., Sinclair, M., VehvilÃinen-Julkunen, K., Beeckman, K., Lotyved, C., & Luybens, A. (2014). Organisational culture in maternity care: A scoping review. *Evidence Based Midwifery*, 12(1), 16–22.

Gabbay, J. (2004). Evidence based guidelines or collectively constructed mindlines? Ethnographic study of knowledge management in primary care. *BMJ*, 329(30), e 1013.

Gillen, P., Sinclair, M., & Kernohan, G. (2008). *The nature and manifestations of bullying in midwifery*. Ulster: University of Ulster. https://www.researchgate.net/publication/265454161_The_nature_and_manifestations_of_bullying_in_midwifery

Glaser, E. (2015). *The Cult of Natural Childbirth Has Gone too Far*. guardian.com. https://www.theguardian.com/commentisfree/2015/mar/05/natural-childbirth-report-midwife-musketeers-morcambe-bay

Goffman, E. (1963). *Stigma. Notes on the Management of Spoiled Identity*. Prentice Hall.

Goodwin, S., & Huppatz, K. E. (2010). The good mother in theory and research: An overview. In S. Goodwin & K. Huppatz (Eds.), *The Good Mother: Contemporary Motherhoods in Australia* (pp. 1–24). Sydney University Press.

Greenfield, M., Payne-Gifford, S., & McKenzie, G. (2021). Between a rock and a hard place: Considering "freebirth" during Covid-19. *Frontiers in Global Women's Health*, 0, 2, 603744. doi: 10.3389/fgwh.2021.603744

Holten, L., & de Miranda, E. (2016). Women's motivations for having unassisted childbirth or high-risk homebirth: An exploration of the literature on 'birthing outside the system'. *Midwifery*, 38, 55–62. doi: 10.1016/j.midw.2016.03.010

Hoschschild, A. (1983). *The Managed Heart. Commercialization of Human Feeling*. University of California Press.

Hunter, B. (2004). Conflicting ideologies as a source of emotion work in midwifery. *Midwifery*, 20(3), 261–272.

Hunter, B. (2005). Emotion work and boundary maintenance in hospital-based midwifery. *Midwifery*, 21(3), 253–266.

Hunter, B. (2010). Mapping the emotional terrain of midwifery: What can we see and what lies ahead? *International Journal of Work Organisation and Emotion*, 3(3), 253–269.

Hunter, B., Fenwick, J., Sidebotham, M., & Henley, J. (2019). Midwives in the United Kingdom: Levels of burnout, depression, anxiety and stress and associated predictors. *Midwifery*, 79. doi: 102526.10.1016/j.midw.2019.08.008

Hunter, B., Henley, J., Fenwick, J., Sidebotham, M., & Pallant, J. (2018). *Work, Health and Emotional Lives of Midwives in the United Kingdom: The UK WHELM study*. Cardiff: Cardiff University. https://www.rcm.org.uk/media/2924/work-health-and-emotional-lives-of-midwives-in-the-united-kingdom-the-uk-whelm-study.pdf

Hunter, M., Smythe, E., & Spence, D. (2018). Confidence: Fundamental to midwives providing labour care in freestanding midwifery-led units. *Midwifery*, 66, 176–181. doi: 10.1016/j.midw.2018.08.016

Hunter, B., & Warren, L. (2013). *Investigating Resilience in Midwifery: Final Report*. Cardiff: Cardiff University. https://orca.cf.ac.uk/61594/1/Investigating%20resilience%20 Final%20report%20oct%202013.pdf

Hunter, B., & Warren, L. (2014). Midwives' experiences of workplace resilience. *Midwifery*, 30(8), 926–934.

ICM. (2014). *Core Document Philosophy and Model of Midwifery Care*. The Hague: ICM. https://www.internationalmidwives.org/assets/files/definitions-files/2018/06/eng-philosophy-and-model-of-midwifery-care.pdf

ICM. (2021). *Building the Enabling Environment for Midwives: A Call to Action for Policymakers*. The Hague: International Confederation of Midwives. https://internationalmidwives.

org/assets/files/general-files/2021/07/11061-eng_icm-enabling-environment-policy-brief_v1.1_20210629.pdf

Jameton, A. (1984). *Nursing Practice: The Ethical Issues*. Prentice Hall.

Jordan, R., & Farley, C. L. (2008). The confidence to practice midwifery: Preceptor influence on student self-efficacy. *Journal of Midwifery & Women's Health*, 53(5), 413–420. doi: 10.1016/j.jmwh.2008.05.001

King's Fund. (2020). *The Courage of Compassion: Supporting Nurses and Midwives to Deliver High-Quality Care*. London: King's Fund. https://www.kingsfund.org.uk/sites/default/files/2020-09/The%20courage%20of%20compassion%20full%20report_0.pdf

Kirkham, M., Stapleton, H., Curtis, P., & Thomas, G. (2002). Stereotyping as a professional defence mechanism. *British Journal of Midwifery*, 10(9), 549–552. doi: 10.12968/bjom.2002.10.9.10609

Kotaska, A. (2011). Guideline-centered care: A two-edged sword. *Birth*, 38(2), 97–98. doi: 10.1111/j.1523–536X.2011.00469.x

Kouzes, J., & Posner, B. (2011). *The Five Practices of Exemplary Leadership* (2nd ed.). The Leadership Challenge Series: Pfeiffer.

Leap, N. (1997). Making sense of horizontal violence in midwifery. *British Journal of Midwifery*, 5(11), 689. doi: 10.12968/bjom.1997.5.11.689

Lewis, L., & Hauck, Y. (2018). Three perspectives on immersion in water for labour and birth. *Women and Birth*, 31, S32. doi: 3110.1016/j.wombi.2018.08.098

Liberati, E., Tarrant, C., Willars, J., Draycott, T., Winter, C., Chew, S., & Dixon-Woods, M. (2019). How to be a very safe maternity unit: An ethnographic study. *Social Science & Medicine* , 223, 64–72.

Link, B. G., & Phelan, J. C. (2001). Conceptualizing stigma. *Annual Review of Sociology*, 27(1), 363–385. doi: 10.1146/annurev.soc.27.1.363

McKenzie, G., & Montgomery, E. (2021). Undisturbed physiological birth: Insights from women who freebirth in the United Kingdom. *Midwifery*, 101, 103042. doi: 10.1016/j.midw.2021.103042

Miller, Abalos, E., Chamillard, M., Ciapponi, A., Colaci, D., ComandÃ, D., Diaz, V., Geller, S., Hanson, C., Langer, A., Manuelli, V., Millar, K., Morhason-Bello, I., Castro, C., Pileggi, V., Robinson, N., Skaer, M., Souza, J., Vogel, J., & Althabe, F. (2016). Beyond too little, too late and too much, too soon: A pathway towards evidence-based, respectful maternity care worldwide. *Lancet*, 388(10056), 2176–2192. doi: 10.1016/S0140–6736(16)31472-6

Nembhard, I. M., & Edmondson, A. C. (2006). Making it safe: The effects of leader inclusiveness and professional status on psychological safety and improvement efforts in health care teams. *Journal of Organizational Behavior*, 27(7), 941–966. doi: 10.1002/job.413

NHS England. (2016). *Better Births: Improving Outcomes of Maternity Services in England*. A Five Year Forward View for maternity care. https://www.england.nhs.uk/wp-content/uploads/2016/02/national-maternity-review-report.pdf

NICE. (2017). *Intrapartum Care for Healthy Women and Babies*. NICE. https://www.nice.org.uk/guidance/cg190/resources/intrapartum-care-for-healthy-women-and-babies-pdf-35109866447557

Nicholls, & Webb. (2006). What makes a good midwife? An integrative review of methodologically diverse research. *Journal of Advanced Nursing*, 56(4), 414–429. doi: 10.1111/j.1365–2648.2006.04026.x

O'Donovan, R., & McAuliffe, E. (2020a). Exploring psychological safety in health-care teams to inform the development of interventions: Combining observational, survey and interview data. *BMC Health Services Research*, 20(1), 810. doi: 10.1186/s12913-020-05646-z

O'Donovan, R., & McAuliffe, E. (2020b). A systematic review exploring the content and outcomes of interventions to improve psychological safety, speaking up and voice behaviour. *BMC Health Services Research*, 20(1), 101. doi: 10.1186/s12913-020-4931-2

Ortashi, O., Virdee, J., Hassan, R., Mutrynowski, T., & Abu-Zidan, F. (2013). The practice of defensive medicine among hospital doctors in the United Kingdom. *BMC Medical Ethics*, 14(1). doi: 10.1186/1472-6939-14-42

Pollard, K. (2011). How midwives' discursive practices contribute to the maintenance of the status quo in English maternity care. *Midwifery*, 27(5), 612–619.

RCM. (2016). *Why Midwives Leave Revisited*. London: RCM. https://www.proquest.com/openview/914f52ff00a17d34da28f892b2d4985d/1.pdf?pq-origsite=gscholar&cbl=506295https

RCM. (2018). *State of Maternity Services Report 2018 in England*. London: RCM. https://www.rcm.org.uk/media/2373/state-of-maternity-services-report-2018-england.pdf

Reitsma, A., Simioni, J., Brunton, G., Kaufman, K., & Hutton, E. K. (2020). Maternal outcomes and birth interventions among women who begin labour intending to give birth at home compared to women of low obstetrical risk who intend to give birth in hospital: A systematic review and meta-analyses. *The Lancet*, 21(100319). https://doi.org/10.1016/j.eclinm.2020.100319

Renfrew, M., McFadden, A., Bastos, M., Campbell, J., Channon, A., Cheung, N., Silva, D., Downe, S., Kennedy, H., Malata, A., McCormick, F., Wick, L., & Declercq, E. (2014). Midwifery and quality care: Findings from a new evidence-informed framework for maternal and newborn care. *Lancet*, 384(9948), 1129–1145. doi: 10.1016/S0140-6736(14)60789-3

Robertson, J. H., & Thomson, A. M. (2016). An exploration of the effects of clinical negligence litigation on the practice of midwives in England: A phenomenological study. *Midwifery*, 33, 55–63. doi: 10.1016/j.midw.2015.10.005

Robinson, A. (2012). The role of consultant midwife: An exploration of the expectations, experiences and intricacies. Doctoral Thesis: University of Southampton.

Rock, L. (2007). The good mother vs. the other mother: The girl-mom. *Journal of the Motherhood Initiative for Research and Community Involvement*, 9(1), 20–28.

Smith, J. (2021). *Nurturing Maternity Staff: How to Tackle Trauma, Stress and Burnout to Create a Positive Working Culture in the NHS*. Pinter & Martin.

Sullivan, K., Lock, L., & Homer, C. S. E. (2011). Factors that contribute to midwives staying in midwifery: A study in one area health service in New South Wales, Australia. *Midwifery*, 27(3), 331–335. doi: 10.1016/j.midw.2011.01.007

Thompson, S., Nieuwenhuijze, M., Low, L., & de Vries, R. (2016). Exploring Dutch midwives' attitudes to promoting physiological childbirth: A qualitative study. *Midwifery*, 42, 67–73. doi: 10.1016/j.midw.2016.09.019

Walsh, D. (2007). *Improving Maternity Services: Small Is Beautiful – Lessons from a Birth Centre*. Radcliffe Publishing.

West, M., Collins, B., Eckhert, R., & Chowla, R. (2017). *Caring to Change: How Compassionate Leadership Can Stimulate Innovation in Health Care*. London: The King's Fund. https://www.kingsfund.org.uk/publications/caring-change

West, M., Eckert, R., Steward, K., & Pamore, B. (2014). *Developing Collective Leadership for Health Care.* London: King's Fund. https://www.kingsfund.org.uk/sites/default/files/field/field_publication_file/developing-collective-leadership-kingsfund-may14.pdf

White Ribbon Alliance. (2011). *Respectful Maternity Care: The Universal Rights of Childbearing Women.* Washington: White Ribbon Alliance.

Wier, J. (2017). Protecting the public: An investigation of midwives perceptions of regulation and the regulator. *Midwifery*, 52, 57–63. doi: 10.1016/j.midw.2017.06.001

Wieringa, S. (2017). Has evidence-based medicine ever been modern? A Latour-inspired understanding of a changing EBM. *Journal of Evaluation in Clinical Practice*, 23(5), 964–970. doi: 10.1111/jep.12752

Woodward, S. (2022). *Maternity in the Spotlight: Patient Safety Now.* https://www.all4maternity.com/maternity-in-the-spotlight-patient-safety-now/

APPENDICES

Appendix 1

TABLE A.1 Participant demographics

Sex	
Female	44
Male	1
	45
Age	
18–24	1
25–34	11
35–44	19
46–54	8
>55	5
	44
Ethnicity	
British African-Caribbean	1
White British	39
White Welsh	2
White Irish	2
White American	1
	45
Region	
North East England	1
North West England	8
Yorkshire and Humber	4

DOI: 10.4324/9781003265443-8

TABLE A.1 Participant demographics (Continued)

Sex	
East Midlands	3
West Midlands	2
Greater London	8
East of England	4
South East England	8
South West England	4
Wales	2
Northern Ireland	1
Scotland	0
	45
Education	
Diploma	4
Degree	24
Postgraduate certificate	3
Master's	12
PhD	2
	45
Year's qualified	
<2	2
2–5	5
6–10	14
11–20	16
>20	7
>30	1
	45
Employment status	
Full-time	32
Part-time	12
Bank	1
	45
Current Clinical Band	
Band 5	2
Band 6	21
Band 7	14
Band 8	5
Other	3
	45
Job role	
Hospital	
Rotational midwife	4
Core midwife Labour Ward	6
Coordinator (shift leader)	2
Community	
Community midwife	8

Sex	
Integrated midwife (community and birth centre)	2
Birth centre	5
Homebirth Team Leader	4
Community Manager	1
Across all settings	
Specialist (i.e. mental health)	5
Supervisor	1
Consultant Midwife	4
Other	
Research	1
Education	2
	45
Those with additional roles	
Secondary	7
Tertiary	3
	10
Type of additional role	
Supervisor	4
Specialist	1
Research	1
	6

Appendix 2

TABLE A.2 Range of alternative birthing decisions reported by study participants with acronym key

BROAD decisions

Declining vaginal examinations during labour

Declining postdates induction of labour (IOL)
Declining recommended IOL for 'risk' factors i.e. IVF pregnancy, >40 years old, previous caesarean
Declining antenatal screening/scans
Declining all monitoring during labour
Freebirth
HOSPITAL
Hospital: Declining antibiotics in labour for GBS+ or PRSOM
Hospital: Declining augmentation for PSROM
Hospital: WVBAC (with telemetry)
Hospital: WVBAC – declining CEFM
Hospital: VBAC3
Hospital: Declining recommended medical interventions (not emergency)
Hospital: Declining medical interventions in emergency situations
Hospital: Twin waterbirth

TABLE A.2 Range of alternative birthing decisions reported by study participants with acronym key (Continued)

BROAD decisions

Hospital: Physiological third stage – PET
Hospital: Breech births outside of guidelines
Hospital: Waterbirth-gestational diabetes-no CEFM
HOMEBIRTH
Homebirth: >40 years old
Homebirth: VBAC
Homebirth: VBAC2
Homebirth: VBAC postdates
Homebirth: Water VBAC
Homebirth: Grand multipara P5–P10
Homebirth: PSROM > 72 hours
Homebirth: GBS+
Homebirth: Diabetes (Type 1 (n = 1) or GDM (n = 3)
Homebirth: Polyhydramnios
Homebirth: Hypothyroidism
Homebirth: Mental health needs
Homebirth: Blood clotting disorder
Homebirth: Epilepsy
Homebirth: Blood-borne virus
Homebirth: Low iron levels
Homebirth: Raised BMI > 35
Homebirth: Raised BMI > 40
Homebirth: Raised BMI > 50
Homebirth: Breech
Homebirth: Twin breech
Homebirth: Twin waterbirth
Homebirth: Twins
Homebirth: Previous history of PPH's
Homebirth: Previous history of shoulder dystocia
Homebirth: Previous history of 3rd-degree tear
Homebirth: Unusual locations
Homebirth: Declining a recommendation of transfer for meconium liquor
Homebirth: Declining transfer for PPH
Homebirth: Declining transfer for stalled second stage of labour
Homebirth: Declining transfer to hospital during prolonged third stage (>3 hours)
BIRTH CENTRE
Birth centre: Outside of 'criteria' (unspecified)
Birth centre: >40 years old
Birth centre: Blood clotting disorder
Birth centre: Antidepressant medication
Birth centre: Gestational diabetes
Birth centre: Waterbirth GBS+
Birth centre: Raised BMI > 35
Birth centre: Raised BMI > 40
Birth centre: VBAC no CEFM
Birth centre: Breech

Acronyms

AMU	Alongside maternity unit (birth centre within hospital grounds)
BMI	Body mass index
CEFM	Continuous electronic fetal monitoring
COC	Continuity of carer
FMU	Free standing maternity unit (birth centre that is situated away from the hospital)
GBS/GBS+	Group B streptococcus
IOL	Induction of labour
MDT	Multi-disciplinary team
OU	Obstetric unit/hospital
P1/P2/P3 etc.	Number of births the woman has had
PET	Pre-eclampsia toxaemia
PPH	Post-partum haemorrhage
PRSOM:	Prolonged rupture of membranes (definitions vary between 12 and 48 hours)
RCM	Royal College of Midwives
RCOG	Royal College of Obstetricians and Gynaecologists
SOM	Supervisor of Midwives
SROM	Spontaneous rupture of membranes
VBAC	Vaginal birth after caesarean section
	VBAC2 Vaginal birth after two caesarean sections
	VBAC3 Vaginal birth after three caesarean sections
	WVBAC Water vaginal birth after caesarean section
	HVBAC Homebirth after caesarean section
	HWVBAC Home waterbirth after caesarean section
VE	vaginal examination

Appendix 3

TABLE A.3 Typology of the midwives' experiences within their micro, meso, and macro workplace contexts

Model	Personal level	Immediate team	Wider team; management, obstetrics, MDT	Broader organisational context	Participants
1. Stigmatised practice	Normal practice for the individual, but is isolated, marginalised and stigmatised. Experienced negative reprisals and punitive action.	Unsupported by immediate team generally (might have one/two good relationships). Frequent conflicts and arguments.	Little support from MDT, or senior staff or management. Frequent conflict/battle when facilitating women's choices. Fears/experiences reprisals/punitive actions.	Little or no pathways or processes, poor or no leadership for women's choices. Hierarchal and patriarchal working culture and structure. Toxic culture for the midwife.	Leanne, Georgina, Beatrice
2. Deviant practice [lone ranger]	Normal practice for the individual, but is isolated, a 'lone ranger'.	Unusual practice within the immediate team, frequent conflicts, but the midwife is generally able to deliver women's choices but at a cost to his/her wellbeing.	Mixed support from MDT, senior staff or management. Frequent disagreements when facilitating women's choices. Although does maintain some level of relationships with wider team.	Little or no pathways or processes. Poor or no leadership for women's choices. Hierarchical and patriarchal working culture and structures. Challenging culture for the midwife.	Alex, Seana, Clara, Ginny, Katie, Margot, Maria, Meg
3. Optimal deviancy [protective teams]	Normal practice for the individual.	Normal practice for the immediate team, supportive relational team working. Collectively, they are mostly able to deliver women's choices.	Mixed support from MDT, or senior staff or management. Frequent conflict/battle when facilitating women's choices. Divisions between community midwives and hospital midwives.	Pathways and process may be present but are not acknowledged by the wider team/trust. Inconsistent leadership. Challenging wider culture for the midwife but has team as a protective factor.	Laura, Kelly, Stella, Zoe, Kate, Jess, Edna, Rose

4. Optimal deviance [respected individually]	Normal practice for the individual.	May or may not work in teams fully supportive of women's alternative choices, but as an individual midwife, s/he is respected and enabled to facilitate women's choices.	Whilst some conflicts may occur, negotiation with MDT, or senior staff or management is feasible. Facilitation of choices may not be culturally embedded, inconsistency present, but as an individual practitioner, s/he is supported to support women's choices.	Pathways and processes are present but inconsistently used across the organisation. Facilitation appears to be dependent upon individual practitioners. Positive leadership. Minimally challenging for the midwife to deliver woman's choices.	Delilah, Jane, Catherine, Susan
5. Sub-optimal normalised practice	Normalised practice for the midwife is in a leadership role.	Faces fears and resistance from midwife caregivers.	May have support from obstetrics and MDT, but may also experience conflicts. Challenges of embedding change across the service.	Role has introduced pathways, processes, liaison with MDT and legal teams. Has supportive leadership. Challenging culture for the midwife, but change is occurring.	Kelly, Rachel, Tracey, Stella, Jenny, Isabel, Hannah, Lauren, Jenna, Trish
6. Optimal normalised practice	Normal practice for the individual.	Normal practice for the immediate team.	Supportive management, senior staff, MDT and leadership. Collaborative working relationships with MDT which are mostly consistent – has 'critical mass'.	Supportive pathways within the Trust, embedded across the maternity service. Processes accessible by women and midwife. Proactive leadership. Wider culture supports woman-centred decision-making, and midwives delivering their care.	Sam, Anna, Caz, Brigid, Becky, Claire, Emily, Kim, Alice, Lucy, Kerry, Amy, James

INDEX

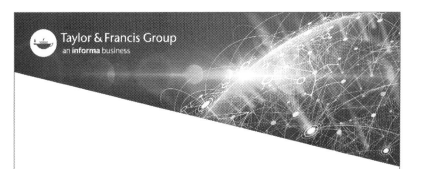

Printed in the United States
by Baker & Taylor Publisher Services